Backpacking Oregon

From the book . . .

Oregon Coast—Seaside to Manzanita *(Trip 1)*

This popular stretch of the Oregon Coast Trail packs a lot of scenic variety in a small area. From beaches and tidepools to dense forests and high viewpoints, this trip has it all.

Rogue River Trail *(Trip 3)*

This wild canyon provides continuously spectacular scenery, waterfalls, [and] unusually abundant wildlife . . . It is unquestionably one of Oregon's most exciting long backpacking trips.

Timberline Trail Loop *(Trip 7)*

. . . probably the most famous footpath in the state . . . The mountain views are stunning, wildflowers choke the meadows, and exceptional side trips abound.

Three Sisters Loop *(Trip 9)*

One of Oregon's greatest long backpacking trips, this route completely circles the Three Sisters, providing ever-changing views of these beautiful siblings . . . A hiker could spend weeks here and never tire of the scenery or run out of places to explore.

Bear Creek Loop *(Trip 19)*

Tucked away in a lesser used corner of the Wallowa Mountains, this loop provides an excellent opportunity for experienced hikers to explore some outstanding country, see plenty of wildlife, and enjoy lonesome trails . . . This trip's main attraction . . . is the spectacular hike along Washboard Ridge, one of the most outstanding ridge walks in Oregon.

Steens Mountain Gorges Loop *(Trip 27)*

The cliffs on the mountain's eastern escarpment drop more than 5500 feet to the flat expanse of Alvord Desert. On the gently sloping west side of the mountain, ice age glaciers carved immense U-shaped gorges that are among the most impressive in the world . . .

Honeycombs Loop *(Trip 29)*

Tucked away on the east side of the Owyhee Reservoir is a land of striking beauty. In the dry canyons of this desert country is a collection of oddly shaped rock pinnacles, towers, and cliffs painted in an array of browns, reds, and oranges.

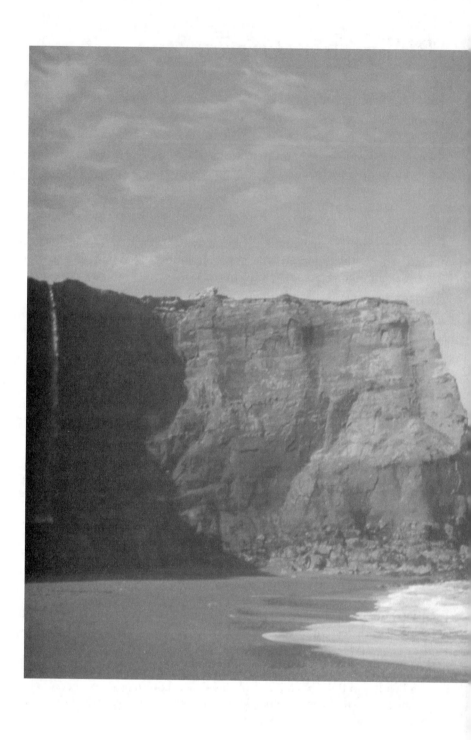

Backpacking
OREGON

From
Rugged Coastline
to Mountain Meadows

Douglas Lorain

🐾 WILDERNESS PRESS ... *on the trail since 1967*

Backpacking Oregon: From Rugged Coastline to Mountain Meadows

1st EDITION September 1999
2nd EDITION May 2007
  3rd PRINTING 2011

Copyright © 2007 and 1999 by Douglas Lorain

Front and back cover photos copyright © 2007 by Douglas Lorain
Photos and maps by the author except as noted
Maps edited by Jaan Hitt and Lisa Pletka
Book design: Jaan Hitt and Larry B. Van Dyke
Book production: Lisa Pletka
Cover design: Lisa Pletka
Book editor: Laura Shauger

ISBN 978-0-89997-441-5

Manufactured in the United States of America

Published by: **Wilderness Press**
                 Keen Communications
                 P.O. Box 43673
                 Birmingham, AL 35243
                 (800) 443-7227; FAX (205) 326-1012
                 info@wildernesspress.com
                 www.wildernesspress.com

Distributed by Publishers Group West

Visit our website for a complete listing of our books and for ordering information.

Cover photos: (front, top) South Sister over Camp Lake, Three Sisters Wilderness
(Trip 9); (front, bottom from left to right) view from Somers Point, Hells Canyon
National Recreation Area (Trip 24); Pleasant Valley, Hells Canyon National
Recreation Area (Trip 26); cliffs near Neahkahnie Mountain (Trip 1);
(back) East Fork Eagle Creek, Wallowa Mountains (Trip 23)

SAFETY NOTICE: Although Wilderness Press and the author have made every
attempt to ensure that the information in this book is accurate at press time, they are
not responsible for any loss, damage, injury, or inconvenience that may occur to
anyone while using this book. You are responsible for your own safety and health
while in the wilderness. The fact that a trail is described in this book does not mean
that it will be safe for you. Be aware that trail conditions can change from day to day.
Always check local conditions and know your own limitations.

Acknowledgments

The help of many people made this book possible. First of all, I would like to thank the hundreds of wilderness rangers and fellow hikers who provided companionship and trip recommendations.

Special thanks go to the following persons:

For introducing me to backpacking, my parents—Bob and Nancy Lorain.

Occasional hiking partners and/or friends—David Elsbernd, Barbara Fink, Bob Fink, and Glenn Sutton.

From the Nature of the Northwest store—Don Haines, who displayed enormous patience and an uncanny ability to answer questions on virtually any subject.

From the Hells Canyon Preservation Council—Ric Bailey.

From the Mazamas—Keith Mischke.

From the Trails Club of Oregon—Walt Garvin.

Forest Service and BLM personnel, who read drafts or otherwise provided their considerable expertise—Bob Alward, Larry Brandvold, Ray Crist, Leigh Dawson, Mary Emerick, Carole Holly, Dwight Johnson, Janet Kirsch, Don McLennan, Randy Menke, Kirk Metzger, Jacquelyn Oakes, Steve Otoupalik, Mike Ricketts, Robin Rose, John Shipp, Cathi Wilbanks, and Sue Womack.

From Oregon State Parks—Pete Bond.

For generously sharing his experience in publishing—William L. Sullivan.

For her botanical expertise—Christine Ebrahimi.

For her love, support, and the countless other wonderful things she brings to my life—my wife, Becky Lovejoy.

While the contributions and assistance of the persons listed above were invaluable, all of the text, maps, and photos herein are my work and sole responsibility. Any and all omissions, errors, and just plain stupid mistakes are mine.

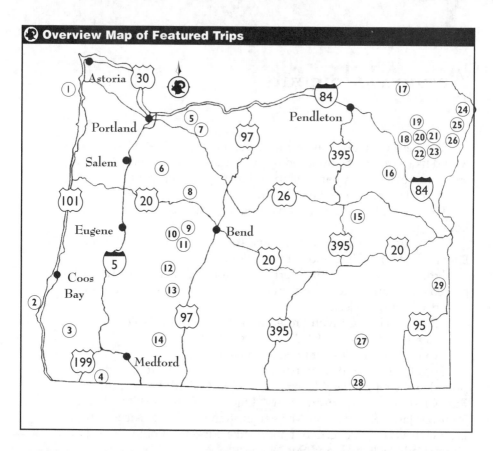

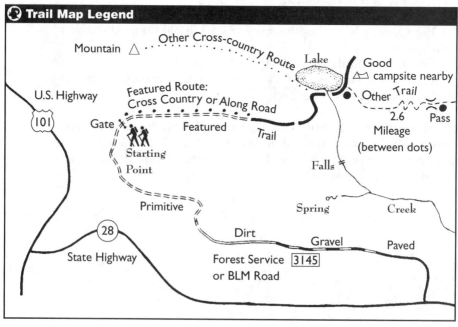

Contents

Featured Trips Summary Chart

| TRIP | (1–10 RATINGS) | | | LENGTH IN: | | ELEV | SHUTTLE |
	SCENERY	SOLITUDE	DIFFICULTY	DAYS	MILES	GAIN	MILEAGE
Trip (Grouped by Typically Best Month)							
April & May							
1 Oregon Coast—Seaside to Manzanita	8	2	5	4	31	4300	23
3 Rogue River Trail	10	5	4	3–6	40	3700	43
17 Wenaha River Trail	9	6	5	3–4	32	2800	22
25 Snake River Trail	10	7	8	4–5	41	6000	N/A
26 Hells Canyon Bench "High"Trail	10	8	8	5–8	63	14,900	46
29 Honeycombs Loop	9	10	8	2–3	17	3500	N/A
June							
5 Columbia River Gorge Loop	6	5	6	4–5	39	6900	N/A
24 Hells Canyon Western Rim "Summit" Trail	8	8	5	5–7	53	7400	63
27 Steens Mountain Gorges Loop	10	8	9	2–4	26	4200	N/A
28 Desert Trail—Pueblo Mountains	8	9	7	2–3	22	6500	20
July							
4 Siskiyou Boundary Trail	8	7	5	4	37	8400	25
12 Diamond Peak Loop	8	6	5	3–4	27	3500	N/A
13 North Umpqua–Mount Thielsen Trails	7	6	6	4–5	46	6800	34
15 Strawberry Mountains Traverse	9	6	7	4	35	7600	31
16 Elkhorn Crest Trail	9	6	6	3	28	3000	33
18 Minam River Loop	7	6	7	3–6	35	5300	N/A
19 Bear Creek Loop	8	8	8	3–6	39	6300	N/A
22 Southern Wallowas Traverse	9	6	8	4–5	40	9400	42
23 East Eagle–Imnaha Loop	10	4	6	5–6	39	7900	N/A
August							
6 Bull of the Woods Loop	6	7	6	3–5	29	6000	N/A
7 Timberline Trail Loop	10	2	7	3–5	41	8600	N/A
8 Mount Jefferson Wilderness Traverse	10	3	6	4–6	44	6400	76
9 Three Sisters Loop	10	2	6	5–6	55	8200	N/A
10 Separation Creek Loop	6	7	6	4–6	42	4700	N/A
14 Sky Lakes Traverse	7	4	5	3–4	31	3600	41
20 Lostine–Minam Loop	9	4	6	4–6	43	8700	N/A
21 Wallowa River Loop	10	2	7	4–5	36	7100	N/A
September							
2 Oregon Coast—Bandon to Port Orford	8	7	4	3–4	29	600	27
11 Mink Lake Area	7	4	3	3	24	1600	16

Preface

Authors of guidebooks face a dilemma. Without dedicated supporters the wilderness would never be protected in the first place. The best and most enthusiastic advocates are those who have actually visited the land, often with the help of a guidebook. On the other hand, too many boots can also be destructive. It is the responsibility of every visitor to tread lightly on the land and to speak out strongly for its preservation.

It is often overlooked that even land officially protected as wilderness needs continued citizen involvement. Issues like use restrictions, grazing rights, mining claims, horse damage, and entry fees all continue to present challenges. Remember you own this land. Treat it with respect and get involved in its management.

To their credit, almost every agency official who reviewed this material stressed the need for hikers to leave no trace of their visit. The author believes the time has come for us to go beyond the well-known "no trace" principles. It must be our goal to leave behind a landscape that not only shows no trace of our presence but is actually in better shape than before we arrived. Here are some guidelines:

- Obviously, be scrupulous to leave no litter of your own. Even better, remove any litter left by others (blessedly little these days).

- Do some minor trail maintenance as you hike. Kick rocks off the trail, remove limbs and debris, and drain water from the path to reduce mud and erosion. Major trail maintenance problems, such as large blowdowns or washouts, should be reported to the land managers so they can concentrate their limited dollars where those are most needed.

- *Always* camp in sites that either are compacted from years of previous use or can easily accommodate a tent without being damaged (sand, gravel bars, and densely wooded areas are best). Never camp on fragile meadow vegetation or beside lakes or streams. If you see camps being established in inappropriate places, be proactive. Place a few limbs or rocks over the area to discourage further use, scatter "horse apples," and remove fire-scarred rocks. Report those who ignore the rules to rangers (or offer to help the offenders move to a better location).

- *Never* feed wildlife and encourage others to do likewise.

- *Do not* build campfires. This holds doubly true for desert areas, where there is little fuel anyway. The author has backpacked thousands of miles in the last 10 years and has built just one fire (and that was only in an emergency). You simply don't need a fire to have a good time, and it is damaging to the land. When you discover a fire ring in an otherwise pristine area, scatter the rocks and cover the fire pit to discourage its use.

- Leave *all* of the following at home: soap—even biodegradable soap pollutes; pets—even well-mannered pets are instinctively seen as predators by wildlife; anything loud; and any outdated attitudes you may have about going out to "conquer" the wilderness.

A Word About Horses

Horses have been a symbol of the American West for hundreds of years. There is something very romantic about seeing horses on the trail. That romance quickly fades, however, when viewing what horses leave behind. The damage done to trails, meadows, and campsites by a single string of horses is *significantly* greater than that done by 100 or more backpackers. Trails are turned into muddy quagmires and rapidly eroded. After dry spells, hikers must contend with clouds of dust on any trail frequented by horses. Camps are trampled, smelly, and soiled by piles of manure. Meadows are chewed to pieces by grazing equines. The list goes on and on.

In response to these problems, land managers are belatedly starting to impose restrictions. Group sizes for parties with livestock are being limited, alternate "horse only" trails are being constructed (often at great expense), and there are restrictions on where horses can camp and graze. Some trails have been closed to horses altogether—and the positive results on the land are obvious and miraculous.

Responsible horse packers (and despite evidence to the contrary, these are the majority) who want to continue to use trails must make a greater effort to reduce their impact. Keep groups *as small as possible*. Scatter manure in the woods away from camping areas. Keep horse strings on one path instead of parallel paths that create "braided" trails and erosion channels. Graze only where grass is abundant—bringing pelletized food is always preferable. Most importantly, *police your own* by reporting and ostracizing those irresponsible horse owners who create a disproportionate share of the problem. If not stopped, these people will eventually interfere with your own ability to use and enjoy the wilderness.

One of the easiest and best ways to reduce horse impact is to keep trails closed to horses, each year, until the tread has dried and hardened. Doing so significantly reduces the problems of mud and erosion. Keeping horses out for as little as two weeks from the typical opening date for hikers makes a huge difference. To the author's knowledge, however, no wilderness in Oregon currently uses this simple and effective management tool. Given the time and energy spent on reducing the impact of *hikers*, this glaring blind spot is difficult to understand.

The future ability of *all* visitors to enjoy the freedom and beauty of the wilderness depends on how we behave in the backcountry today. Our children and grandchildren deserve nothing less than our best efforts to protect these treasures for the future.

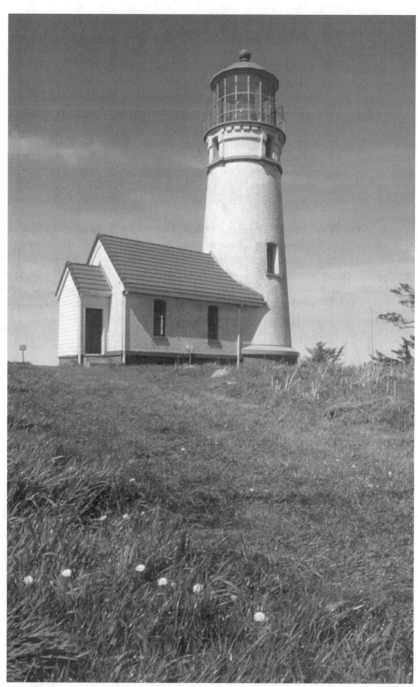

Cape Blanco Lighthouse (Trip 2)

A Word about the Second Edition

Thanks to the enthusiastic response of hikers in every corner of the state, *Backpacking Oregon* now goes proudly into its second edition, bigger and better than ever. Fans of the first edition will recognize the familiar user-friendly format as well as most of the trips, but they will also find three exceptional new outings to explore.

All but one of the outstanding trips described in the first edition have been retained—extensive damage from the 2002 Biscuit Fire has made the Kalmiopsis Loop unattractive and difficult to hike. Reader suggestions have caused major revisions in another trip, the Bull of the Woods Loop, which make this hike more compact and easier to follow. But readers will probably be most excited by the three new trips. Like many of the old trips, these new adventures in the Wallowa Mountains and Three Sisters Wilderness visit isolated parts of Oregon that are unfamiliar to many. In fact, these loop trips have never been fully described in any guidebook. In addition to helping backpackers find solitude, the new outings are very scenic and fun to hike. Awaiting your discovery along these trails are impressive old-growth forests, secluded wilderness lakes, a long alpine ridgeline with spectacular views, and a deep wilderness canyon carved by a sparkling, clear river. In addition to the new trips, the original hikes have been carefully updated to reflect changes in trail conditions, roads, telephone numbers, administrative rules, and the like.

Perhaps this edition's most noticeable change, and the one that readers have asked for more consistently than any other, is the full-color photography. The goal of these pictures is, not only to dazzle you with the spectacular scenery found in the Oregon backcountry, but to provide a more realistic representation of a given trip's terrain so you can better see if it fits your outdoor tastes and preferences.

I invite all readers, whether new to hiking and this book or already wearing boots worn ragged from years of backpacking, to use this second edition as a guide to many years of great adventures in the wildlands of Oregon. I hope you enjoy touring these trails as much as I did. Please feel free to contact me, in care of Wilderness Press, with your suggestions and updates so that this book can continue to be the best and most accurate backpacking guide to the Beaver State.

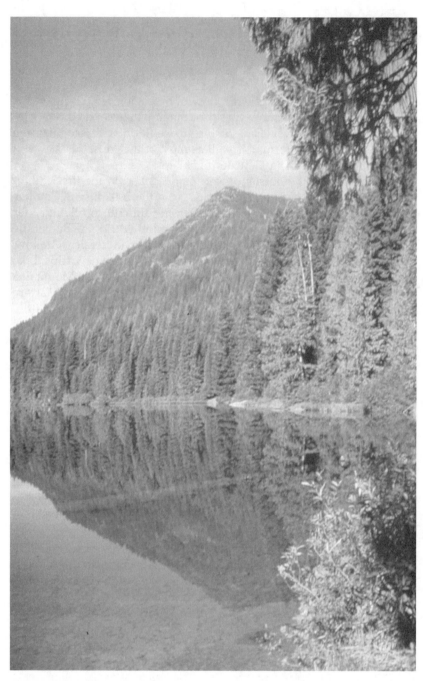

Battle Ax over Elk Lake (Trip 6)

Introduction

Here's the scenario: You're an avid backpacker dreaming of your annual vacation away from the rat race. You've read the magazines, pored over the guidebooks, and seen all the famous pictures. After careful consideration, you've decided on a hike through the spectacular lakes and white granite peaks of California's Sierra Nevada. Or perhaps it's Arizona's Grand Canyon that draws your attention, or British Columbia's wild Pacific Coast, or the canyon country of southern Utah. Months in advance you book reservations to get one of the few available permits. Then you plunk down hundreds of dollars for a plane ticket or get in your car and drive for several days to reach your destination. Once there, you're faced with crowds of other admiring backpackers who have come from all over the world to enjoy the same famous scenery. You still have a great vacation, but naturally you resent all the headaches.

Take heart. What many people apparently don't realize is that much the same scenery can be found in Oregon without the accompanying hassles. Oregon has remarkable geographic diversity. You can hike wild beaches, enjoy colorful desert canyonlands, walk amid stunning granite peaks, relax in wildflower meadows, circle glacier-clad mountains, and explore trails through the deepest river canyon on the continent—all in one state! To be sure, all those more famous places deserve their reputations for beauty. But what Oregon has to offer is also spectacular, and, at its best, just as grand. So if your purpose is to brag about how you've been to some well-known place, then, by all means, fight the crowds in Yosemite or wherever. But if your goal is to simply enjoy glorious scenery with fewer headaches, then consider the trails in Oregon.

There are many ways to see and appreciate the beauty of Oregon. Many parts of the state can be seen just as easily (sometimes more efficiently) by dayhikes, rafting trips, bicycle tours, or even from your car. The focus of this book, however, is on the best ways for backpackers to see the state. After many years and tens of thousands of trail miles, the author has listed what he believes to be Oregon's very best backpacking trips. The focus is on longer trips—from three days to two weeks. These are beyond a simple weekend outing, but they make terrific vacations, and give you enough time to fully appreciate the scenery. Best of all, you'll have the chance to get to know and love the country.

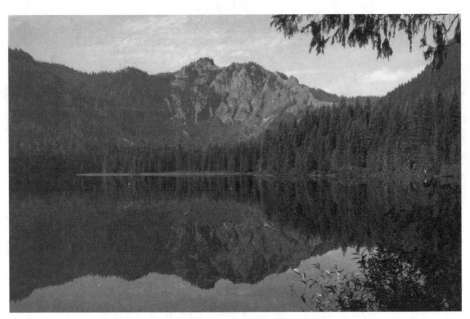

Bear Creek at Dobbin Trail ford, Wallowa Mountains (Trip 19)

HOW TO USE THIS GUIDE

Each featured trip begins with an information box that provides a quick overview of the hike's vital statistics and important features. This lets you rapidly narrow down your options based on your preferences, your abilities, how many days you have available, and the time of year.

SCENERY: This is the author's subjective opinion of the trip's overall scenic quality, on a 1 (an eyesore) to 10 (drop-dead-gorgeous) scale. This rating is based on the author's personal biases in favor of flowers, photogenic views, and clear streams. If your tastes run more toward lush forests or good fishing, then your own rating may be quite different. Also keep in mind that the rating is a *relative* one. *All* the featured trips are beautiful, and if they were somehow transplanted to, say, Nebraska, would justifiably draw crowds of admirers.

SOLITUDE: Since solitude is one of the things backpackers are seeking, it helps to know roughly how much company you can expect. This rating is also on a 1 (bring stilts to see over the crowds) to 10 (just you and the juncos) scale. Of course, even on a trip rated as a 9 or 10, there's always an outside chance you'll end up plagued by a pack of wild Cub Scouts.

DIFFICULTY: This is yet another subjective judgment by the author. The rating is intended to warn you away from the most difficult outings if you're not in shape to try them. The scale is only *relative to other* *backpacking trips.* Most Americans would find even the easiest back-packing trip to be a very strenuous undertaking. So this scale of 1 (bare-ly leave the La-Z-Boy) to 10 (the Ironman Triathlon) is only for people already accustomed to backpacking.

MILEAGE: This is the total mileage of the recommended trip in its *most basic form* (with no side trips). The author, however, has never seen the point of a "bare bones," Point A to Point B kind of trip. After all, if you're going to go, you may as well explore a bit. Thus, for most trips there is also a *second* mileage number (in parentheses below) that includes distances for recommended side trips. These side trips are also shown on the maps and included in the "Possible Itinerary" section. (**Note:** Some exact mileages were not available, especially for cross-country routes. The mileage shown may be only an approximation—based on extrapolation from maps or the author's own pedometer readings.)

ELEVATION GAIN: For many hikers, how far *UP* they go is even more important than the distance. This entry shows the trip's *total* elevation gain, not the *net* gain. As with the mileage section, a second number (in parentheses below) also includes the elevation gain in recommended side trips.

DAYS: This is a *rough* figure for how long it will take the average backpacker to do the trip. It is based on the author's preference for traveling about 10 miles per day. Also considered were the spacing of available campsites and the trip's difficulty. Hard-core hikers may cover as many as 25 miles a day, while others saunter along at 4 or 5 miles per day, a good pace for hikers with children. Most trips can be done in more or fewer days, depending on your preferences and abilities.

SHUTTLE MILEAGE: This is the shortest one-way driving distance between the beginning and the ending trailheads. Be sure to schedule enough time at both ends of your trip to complete the necessary car shuttle.

MAP: Every trip includes a sketch map that is as up-to-date and accurate as possible. As every hiker knows, however, you'll also need a good contour map of the area. This line identifies the best available map(s) for the described trip. All references to USGS maps are for the 7.5' series.

SEASON: There are actually *two* seasonal entries shown for each trip. The first tells you when a trip is usually snow-free enough for hik-ing (which can vary considerably from year to year). The second entry lists the particular time(s) of year when the author thinks the trip is typically at its best (when the flowers peak, the fall colors are at their best, or the mosquitoes have died down, etc.). Unfortunately, the "best" season may also be the most crowded, so you may prefer to visit when conditions aren't as good, but you'll enjoy more solitude.

PERMITS AND RULES: Regulations are changing very rapidly in the Oregon backcountry. Several areas now require backpackers to obtain and carry permits. Managers are also restricting the number of hikers allowed into traditionally crowded locations. These permits were initially free, but cash-strapped agencies will soon charge for them. Generally, you should obtain backcountry permits from the nearest Forest Service ranger station. It is always advisable to call ahead and ask about current restrictions and the need for reservations, since the regulations are constantly changing.

CONTACT: This is the telephone number for the local land agency responsible for this area. Be sure to check on road and trail conditions as well as any new restrictions or permit requirements before your trip.

SPECIAL ATTRACTIONS: This section focuses on attributes of this trip that are rare or outstanding. For example, almost every trip has views, but some have views that are *especially* noteworthy. The same is true of areas with a good chance of seeing wildlife, with excellent fishing, and so on.

PROBLEMS: This is the flip side to the "Special Attractions" section. It lists the trip's special or especially troublesome problems. Expect to see warnings about areas with particularly abundant mosquitoes, poor road access, or limited water.

TIPS, WARNINGS, AND NOTES: Throughout the text are numerous helpful hints and ideas. These all result from the author's experience. A pessimist once said that experience is something you never have until just after you need it. By relying on the hard-won experience of others, these prominently labeled *Tips,* *Warnings,* and *Notes* will hopefully make your trips safer and more enjoyable the *first* time through.

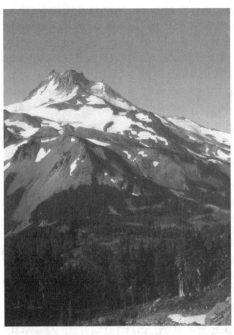

Mount Hood from near Cairn Basin (Trip 7)

POSSIBLE ITINERARY: This is listed at the *end* of each trip. To be used as a planning tool, it includes daily mileages and total elevation gains, as well as recommended side trips. Your own itinerary is likely to be different. Although the author has hiked all the listed trips, most were not done quite as written here. If he were to re-hike the trip, however, he would follow the improved itineraries here.

SAFETY NOTICE

The trips described in this book are long, and often difficult, and some go through remote wilderness terrain. In the event of an emergency, supplies and medical facilities may be several days away. Anyone who attempts these hikes must be experienced in wilderness travel, properly equipped, and in good physical condition. While backpacking is not inherently dangerous, the sport *does* involve risk. Because trail conditions, weather, and hikers' abilities all vary considerably, the author and the publisher cannot assume responsibility for the safety of anyone who takes these hikes. Use plenty of common sense and a realistic appraisal of your abilities so you can enjoy these trips safely.

References to "water" in the text attest only to its availability, not its purity. All backcountry water should be treated before drinking.

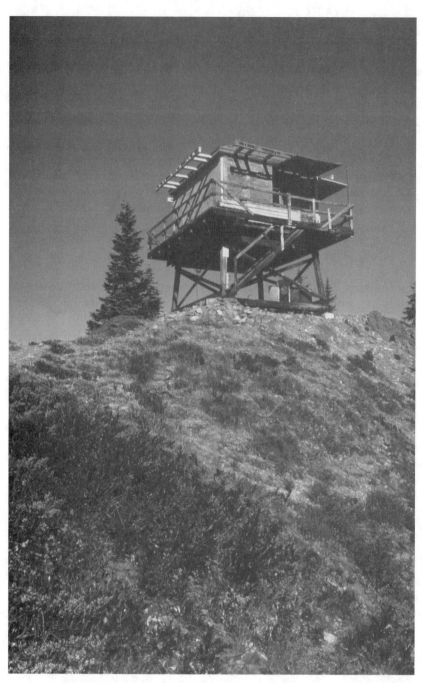

Fire lookout atop Bull of the Woods (Trip 6)

General Tips on
Backpacking in Oregon

This book is not a "how to" guide for backpackers. Anyone contemplating an extended backpacking vacation will (or at least *should*) already know about equipment, the "no trace" ethic, conditioning, how to select a campsite, food, first aid, and all the other aspects of this sport. There are a myriad of excellent books covering these subjects. It is appropriate, however, to discuss some tips and ideas that are specific to Oregon and the Pacific Northwest.

1) Most national forests in Oregon require a trailhead parking pass. In general, a windshield sticker is required for cars parked within 0.25 mile of major developed trailheads. As of 2010, daily permits cost $5, and an annual pass, good in all the forests of Oregon and Washington, was $30 (actually a pretty good deal). The fees are used for trail maintenance, wilderness rangers' pay, and trailhead improvements.

2) The winter's snowpack has a significant effect, not only on when a trail opens, but also on peak wildflower times, peak stream flows, and how long seasonal water sources will be available. You can check the snowpack on about April 1 and note how it compares to normal. This information is available through the local media or by contacting the Snow Survey Office in Portland (503) 414-3270, or go to www.or.nrcs.usda.gov/snow. If the snowpack is significantly above or below average, adjust the trip's seasonal recommendations accordingly.

3) When driving on Oregon's forest roads, keep a wary eye out for log trucks. These scary behemoths often barrel along with little regard for those annoying speed bumps known as passenger cars.

4) An excellent storehouse of maps, books, knowledgeable personnel, and up-to-date information is the Nature of the Northwest store located at 800 NE Oregon Street in Portland; their phone number is (971) 673-2331. This store coordinates recreation data from the Forest Service, BLM, and other land agencies into one central facility. A call or visit here will be well worth your time. They also sell the complete line of Forest Service and BLM maps.

5) This book focuses exclusively on backpacking trips. For dayhikes a different resource is necessary. The best dayhike guidebooks for the state are the 100 Hikes series by William L. Sullivan, published by

Navillus Press. The five-book series covers the state from the coast to eastern Oregon and is indispensable.

6) The Northwest's frequent winter storms create annual problems for trail crews. Early-season hikers should expect to crawl over deadfall and search for routes around slides and flooded riverside trails. Depending on current funding and the trail's popularity, maintenance may not be completed until several weeks after a trail is snow free and officially "open." Unfortunately, this means trail maintenance is often done well after the "best" time to visit. On the positive side, trails are usually less crowded before the maintenance has been completed.

7) For environmentally conscious backpackers, one good solution to the old dilemma of how to dispose of toilet paper is to find a natural alternative. Two excellent options are the large, soft leaves of thimbleberry at lower elevations and the light green lichen that hangs from trees at higher elevations. They're not exactly Charmin soft, but they get the job done.

8) Mid-August is usually the best time for swimming in mountain lakes. Water temperatures (while never exactly tropical) are at their warmest, and the bugs have decreased enough to allow you to dry off in relative peace. A swimsuit makes a good addition to your gear for any trip to the mountains at this time of year, or you can go with a birthday suit in less popular areas.

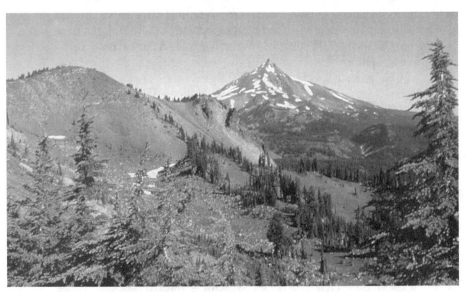

Mount Jefferson and North Cinder Peak from the Pacific Crest Trail to the south (Trip 8)

9) General deer-hunting season in Oregon runs from the first weekend of October to the end of the month or early November. Also, for a week in early to mid-September, Oregon holds a "High Cascades" deer hunt in the wilderness areas of the Cascade Mountains. For safety, anyone planning to travel in the forests during these periods (particularly those doing any cross-country travel) should carry and wear a bright red or orange cap, vest, pack, or other conspicuous article of clothing.

10) Elk hunting season is in late October or, more often, early November. The exact season varies in different parts of the state.

11) Mushrooms are an Oregon backcountry delicacy. Although our damp climate makes it possible to find mushrooms in any season, late August through November is usually best. Where and when the mushrooms can be found varies with elevation, precipitation, and other factors.

Warnings: Mushroom collecting has become a very competitive business. A few people have even been murdered in recent years in disputes over prize locations. Second, make absolutely sure you know your fungi. There are several poisonous species in our forests, and you do not want to make a mistake.

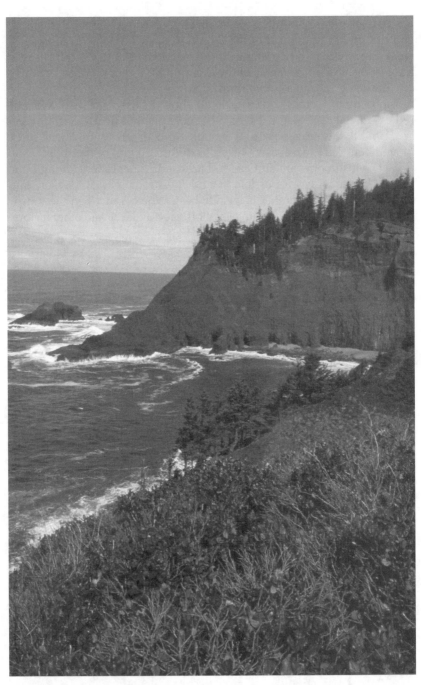

View north from Cape Falcon (Trip 1)

Wild Areas of Oregon

What follows is a general overview of the principal remaining wild areas in the state of Oregon. All of these have at least one backpacking trip in the featured-trips section. Thus, whether you're a desert rat, a mountain man, a canyon lover, or a beach bum, there's a choice of outstanding trips for you.

It is appropriate here to say a few words about Crater Lake. As Oregon's only national park, Crater Lake is probably the best-known scenic attraction in the state. It is also the only major natural wonder for which there is no recommended trip. Construction of the rim road around the lake created one of the most spectacular drives in North America and simultaneously eliminated any chance for developing what would have been one of the most spectacular *hikes* on the continent. Today the park features only short (but very scenic) dayhikes. The only backpacking is through generally viewless forests, well away from the lake, with little to recommend it other than solitude. The best plan is to visit the park (it really is too good to miss), take a dayhike or two, and then head for the longer trails in the nearby Mount Thielsen, Rogue River, or Sky Lakes areas.

OREGON COAST

The Oregon coast is world-famous. Countless thousands of tourists drive up and down this shoreline enjoying some of the continent's best scenery. The coastal highway has also become a popular bicycle tour. Despite this popularity, there are still places suitable for extended backpacking trips along this magnificent stretch of beaches, rocks, cliffs, and coastal forests.

In addition to the scenery, hikers are drawn to the coast's abundant and diverse wildlife. Long before we *Homo sapiens* built summer homes at the beach, it attracted countless other species. Keep an eye out for whales, harbor seals, and sea lions. Tidepools teem with life in a dizzying array of forms and colors. The Oregon coast is especially popular with our feathered friends. The cliffs and offshore rocks here support some 1.2 million nesting birds—more than the coasts of California and Washington *combined*, even though the total shorelines of those two states is almost five times longer. Nesting bird numbers peak from about mid-May to the end of June.

Note: *All offshore rocks are part of a protected wildlife refuge and are strictly off limits to people. Bring binoculars to get a close-up view.*

There are two down sides to coastal hiking. The first, of course, is crowds. Visiting mid-week helps, but the best plan is to hike in the off season. The beach is a great place to visit during a patch of good weather in the winter, and is equally scenic in fall (after Labor Day) or spring (before Memorial Day).

The second drawback to coastal backpacking is the notorious Oregon weather. In winter the chances of three or four consecutive days of good weather are slim. In summer the coast is often socked in by a thick layer of fog (a fact omitted from Chamber of Commerce brochures). Spring and fall are usually better, but rain and wind are always possible.

KLAMATH AND SISKIYOU MOUNTAINS

Most of southwestern Oregon is a jumbled mass of ancient mountains cut by scenic river canyons. These mountains are much older than the better-known Cascades or Wallowas, and their peculiar geology and botany are a large part of their charm. Unique soils and millions of

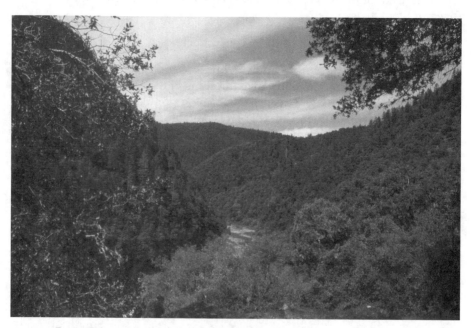

Rogue River Canyon below Blanco Creek (Trip 3)

years of isolation have resulted in Oregon's greatest concentration of rare and unusual plants. This region is truly a botanist's paradise.

The higher Siskiyou Mountains to the east are friendlier terrain for hikers. They feature less steep trails, small lakes, diverse forests, and cooler summer temperatures. Both ranges provide lots of solitude, wildflowers, and surprisingly abundant wildlife.

COLUMBIA RIVER GORGE

Despite its close proximity to a major city and the presence of an interstate freeway, railroads, towns, and dams, much of the Columbia River Gorge remains remarkably wild. Thousands of dayhikers hit the trails here every weekend to see the waterfalls, canyons, lush vegetation, clear streams, and views. By hiking a combination of the area's longer trails, the backpacker can enjoy these same features, with the added benefit of relative solitude. The Gorge is especially beautiful in late spring, when the wildflowers are blooming and the waterfalls are more impressive, and in late October and very early November, when the dogwoods and maples turn color and people are scarce. Summer, on the other hand, is a poor time for a visit, due to crowds and the often hot and muggy conditions at these lower elevations.

The Gorge also has a few hazards. Poison oak is common at elevations below about 1,000 feet. Early-season hikers should expect some trails to be closed due to washouts or landslides. Darkness comes very quickly in these steep canyons, especially in the fall—so make camp early. Finally, even though elevations are relatively low, hikes here usually require a great deal of climbing—since you start near sea level along the Columbia River. Getting to the tops of those cliffs and ridges requires lots of sweat.

WESTERN "OLD" CASCADES

Only a couple of generations ago the western "Old" Cascades were still a vast forested wilderness. Huge old-growth forests, crystal-clear streams, rugged ridges, and small mountain lakes were just some of the treasures that have now been largely replaced by clearcuts and logging roads. Only tiny fragments of the old forests remain, either in isolated preserves or as forested strips near highways or rivers. Exploring the Old Cascades now is best done in the form of dayhikes. Backpackers have the option of hiking longer river trails (usually paralleling roads, such as Trips 36 and 38) or seeking out one of the larger preserves that still have a good sampling of what's left. Two such areas are the Bull of the Woods and Middle Santiam wilderness areas.

Elevations are lower here than in the nearby High Cascades so the trails are free of snow sooner and stay open later. The most attractive times to visit are from mid-June to mid-July, when the rhododendrons bloom, and autumn, with its sprinkling of color and mushrooms. There are no spectacular jagged peaks to admire, but for the spiritual renewal you get from a cathedral-like forest, clear fishing streams, uncrowded trails, and lush vegetation this country is ideal.

Generally off-trail travel is difficult-to-impossible, although the occasional elk or deer path can be followed. Stick to the maintained routes or follow streambeds during the lower water of autumn. Finally, you'll need to bring a good up-to-date map to find trailheads amidst the maze of logging roads.

HIGH CASCADES

Many of the trips in this guide are in the High Cascades—centered around well-known volcanic peaks like Mount Hood, Mount Jefferson, and the Three Sisters. These are the signature mountains of the state, and they deserve their popularity. All feature exceptional scenery, wildflower-filled meadows, and miles of trails. Even backpacking snobs who avoid any trail with the slightest whiff of popularity can't resist doing a classic trip like the Timberline Trail at least once in a lifetime. The peaks in the south part of the range are lower and lack glaciers, but they are also less crowded. Between these peaks, the High Cascades feature great expanses of forests and countless lakes. Fortunately, most of the best areas have been set aside as wilderness, so the backpacker can enjoy many days of scenic travel without the intrusion of roads, chainsaws, or motorbikes.

The ultimate way to experience these mountains is to hike from one end of the state to the other along the Pacific Crest Trail. From Fish Lake (east of Medford) to the Columbia River at Cascade Locks is a total of 380 trail miles (excluding side trips). Most people have neither the time nor the energy to tackle this month-long excursion. A few well-chosen backpacking vacations of 4–10 days, however, can hit all the highlights and provide enough memories to last a lifetime.

Summer in the Oregon Cascades is just about ideal. While you should come prepared for rain, your chances of encountering endless days of wetness are actually rather small, despite all those stories we tell out-of-staters in an effort to keep them out. You should expect rain perhaps one day in four, and it is even possible to go weeks without any rain. Temperatures are usually in the comfortable range (both day and night) with low humidity. Flowers bloom in profusion, and the quiet hiker has a good chance of seeing wildlife. There are no dangerous animals to worry about, since rattlesnakes are found on the east side only at lower elevations, and grizzly bears have been gone for over a century. Even horse flies and deer flies—so abundant in other parts of North America—are rarely a problem in these mountains. The only problems worth mentioning are mosquitoes (particularly in the lake country), and the need to get permits for some areas as land managers slowly try to reduce the impact of too many visitors.

BLUE MOUNTAINS

For the most part, northeastern Oregon's Blue Mountains are a gentle region of rolling mountains, open forests, and enticing meadows. In places, however, subranges with snowy crags and sparkling lakes reach dramatically skyward. Elsewhere, rivers have cut impressive canyons into the lava tablelands. At these special places, the backpacker can enjoy not only grand scenery but also lightly traveled trails.

The Wallowas (see the subsection below) are the best-known mountains in this area, but the Strawberry Mountains and the Elkhorn Range have very similar scenery with only a fraction of the people. Like the Wallowas, these smaller and more compact ranges feature craggy granite peaks, sparkling lakes, meadows ablaze with wildflowers, and wildlife such as elk, bighorn sheep, and mountain goats. *Unlike* in the Wallowas, the hiker won't have to face trails pounded to dust by heavy horse use or compete with hundreds of other hikers for a campsite.

Another uncrowded retreat in these mountains is the Wenaha-Tucannon Wilderness, straddling the border with Washington. This large area is highlighted by the scenic canyons of the Wenaha River and its tributaries. The hike described in Trip 17 follows the length of this lovely fishing stream.

A big advantage for hikers accustomed to the jungles of the western Cascades is the open nature of the forests here. The drier climate means less undergrowth, so cross-country travel is much easier. The weather is also generally better, except for afternoon thunderstorms. Mosquitoes present the usual problems near lakes in July, and rattlesnakes are common in the lower canyons.

WALLOWA MOUNTAINS

Although billed as America's "Little Switzerland," the Wallowa Mountains of northeastern Oregon are actually more similar to California's Sierra Nevada. (That comparison, however, apparently doesn't carry the same marketing appeal.) The mountains are a stunningly beautiful mix of white granite peaks, sparkling lakes and streams, alpine meadows, and attractive forests. Even better, God

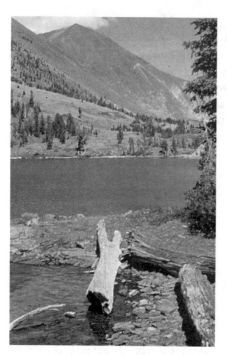

Ice Lake, Wallowa Mountains (Trip 21)

seemingly designed this paradise with the backpacker in mind. The bulk of the most scenic country is beyond the range of dayhikers. For the long-distance hiker, however, the Eagle Cap Wilderness is laced with hundreds of miles of interconnecting trails. Since over 75 percent of all visits are to the Lakes Basin, Aneroid Lake, and Glacier Lake areas, there are many miles of lonesome trails in other areas to explore.

Relative to the region's attributes, the down sides are so minor only a true pessimist could dwell on them. You should, nonetheless, be prepared for crowds in a few areas, mosquitoes near the lakes in July, afternoon thunderstorms, and dusty (and "aromatic") trails due to fairly heavy horse use.

Most of the range's many highlights are within the areas of the described trips. If, like the author, you develop a love for this country and want to see more, there are dozens of additional places to explore. Almost any chosen destination will reward you with beautiful scenery and wonderful memories.

HELLS CANYON

The enormity of Hells Canyon is impossible to describe. It is one of those places both words and photographs seem unable to capture adequately. It must be personally experienced to be properly appreciated. Unlike the heavily forested trails familiar to most Oregonians, the mostly treeless routes here present nonstop great views. The gaping chasm, backed by the snow-capped peaks of Idaho's Seven Devils Mountains, presents an incredible expanse of jaw-dropping scenery. The canyon is also one of the best areas for viewing wildlife in the state. Elk, deer, black bear, coyote, bighorn sheep, mountain goat (on the Idaho side), numerous birds, and various reptiles are all common.

Like the canyon itself, the problems associated with backpacking in Hells Canyon are also on a grand scale. Summer's heat in the shadeless lower canyon is unbearable. Rattlesnakes, ticks, and black widow spiders are all common, and the canyon supports large populations of black bears and mountain lions. Although no one has been attacked, hikers have reported being stalked by lions. Thickets of poison ivy crowd the lower-elevation trails near water. Even the main trails are often rough, steep, and hard to follow, and lesser-used paths may be nothing more than rumors. Access roads (when they exist at all) are typically long, rough, dirt roads that may be impassable for passenger cars, and should generally not be attempted when wet. This is truly the realm of the dedicated adventurer.

Three roughly parallel trails travel the entire north-south length of the canyon. Each is described in the text. Since they are at different elevations, they have different peak seasons. Numerous connecting paths allow for loop trips of almost any length.

Along with the adjoining Wallowa Mountains and Idaho's Seven Devils Mountains, this national treasure has been proposed as a national park and preserve. For more information about this worthwhile idea, contact the Hells Canyon Preservation Council at Box 2768, La Grande, Oregon 97850.

MOUNTAINS OF SOUTHEAST OREGON

Oregon is famous for its dense green forests, rain-soaked valleys, and glacier-clad peaks. Not so well known is that fully one-third of the state is desert. *Brown* is the predominate color of southeastern Oregon, not green. Trees are either scarce or nonexistent. Rain falls infrequently, and glaciers are just a distant memory.

Although the landscape differs from western Oregon, it is at least as scenic. The country is especially appealing to those who prefer open views to the claustrophobic feel of dense forests, and dry weather to overcast and drizzle. The principal attractions for backpackers are the mountain ranges that rise dramatically from the sagebrush plains. These spectacular mountains have water (due to more precipitation at higher elevations), lots of flowers, and views that seem to stretch to eternity. Most of the mountains also have few (if any) people. Wildlife is no more abundant here than elsewhere in Oregon, but the lack of dense vegetation makes it much easier to actually *see* the animals.

The best known and most spectacular mountain is Steens Mountain, with its great glacial gorges and towering snowy cliffs. Other nearby ranges like the Pueblo, Hart, and Trout Creek mountains provide more solitude for those who want to gain a more meaningful distance from the world of crowds and machines. To truly get away from it all, just head off into the seemingly endless sagebrush. A few of the more interesting areas to consider are Beatys Butte, Orejana Canyon, Coyote Lake, Hawk Mountain, Oregon End Table, and Diablo

Mountain. If you can even find these places on the map, you'll be well on your way to your own desert adventure.

Those unaccustomed to desert travel must beware of some unique hazards. Expect rattlesnakes, ticks (*extremely* abundant in spring), long distances between water sources, poorly maintained roads, and few (if any) established trails.

OWYHEE COUNTRY

Hidden in southeastern Oregon near the Idaho border is a land that looks more typical of southern Utah than Oregon. Cutting into the sagebrush plains and mountains of this region are several spectacularly deep slot canyons and colorful rock formations. The cliffs are home to bighorn sheep, while pronghorns and wild horses roam the plateaus. It all adds up to a stunningly scenic land with the added advantage of being a great place to go for solitude. There are *no* crowds here; in fact you are unlikely to see another human being in weeks of hiking.

The isolation creates unique problems requiring extra precautions. The only trails are those traveled by deer or cattle, so at least one group member must be very good with a map and compass (you might consider bringing a GPS device). Many of the "roads" here are very poor, especially if wet, and rarely traveled. Carry plenty of emergency gear in your car—extra food, *lots* of extra water, spare parts and tools, etc. Bring along an especially well-stocked first-aid kit (and, of course, you *are* up-to-date on your first-aid methods and skills, right?). Except for the bottoms of major river canyons, water is very scarce. In addition, the canyon country throughout southeastern Oregon gets extremely hot during the summer season (June to mid-September). Carry *at least* three gallons of water in your car, and a gallon per day when hiking. You should always assume water sources are badly polluted by live-stock—*double treat* all water. The author's preference is to first use iodine, wait, and then filter it.

The above precautions aside, this area is well worth the extra effort to explore. Spring (from late April through May) is especially nice, with wildflowers, cooler temperatures, and more water. To hike the canyons, however, fall is usually better because water levels are lower and you won't have to do as much wading.

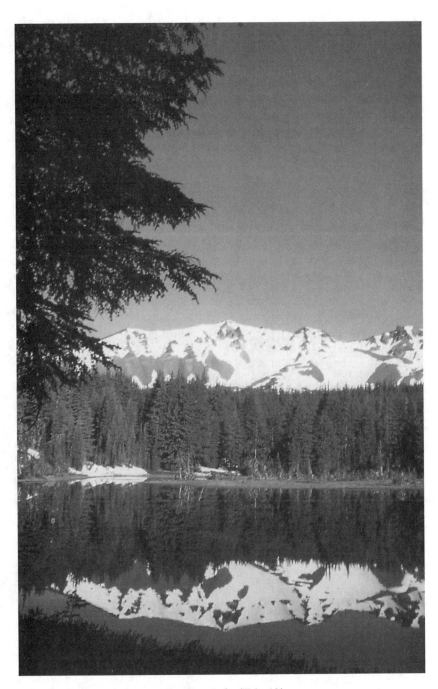

Diamond Peak over Mountain View Lake (Trip 12)

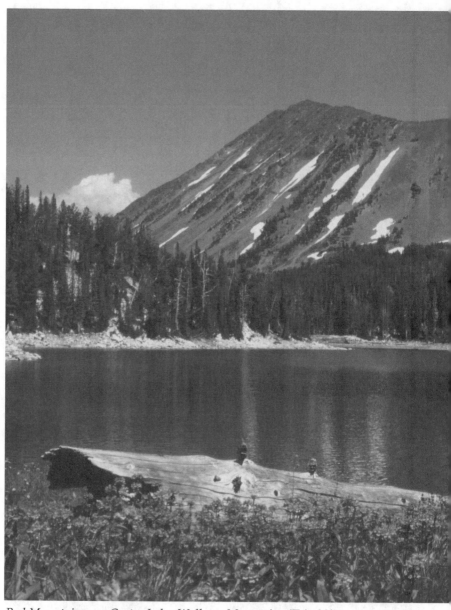

Red Mountain over Crater Lake, Wallowa Mountains (Trip 23)

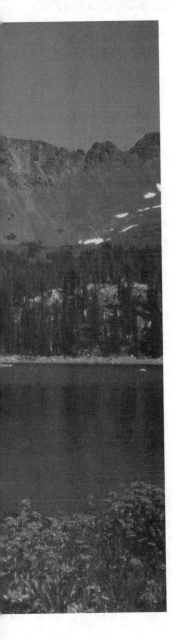

Featured Trips

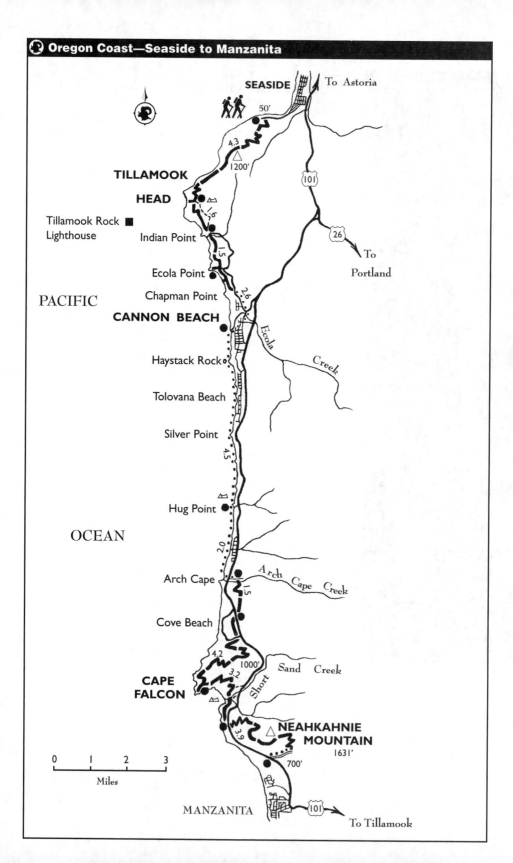

SEASIDE   To Astoria

50'

4.3

1200'

TILLAMOOK

HEAD

Tillamook Rock ■
Lighthouse

Indian Point

1.6

1.5

Ecola Point

Chapman Point

PACIFIC

CANNON BEACH

2.6

Haystack Rock

Ecola

Creek

Tolovana Beach

Silver Point

4.5

OCEAN

Hug Point

2.0

Arch Cape

Arch Cape Creek

1.5

Cove Beach

CAPE
FALCON

4.2

1000'

3.2

Short

Sand   Creek

NEAHKAHNIE
MOUNTAIN

1631'

3.9

700'

0   1   2   3

Miles

MANZANITA   To Tillamook

101

26   To
Portland

1 Oregon Coast— Seaside to Manzanita

RATINGS (1–10)			MILES	ELEVATION GAIN	DAYS	SHUTTLE MILEAGE
Scenery	Solitude	Difficulty				
8	2	5	31	4300	4	23

MAP Use *100 Oregon Coast & Coast Range Hikes* book

USUALLY OPEN All year

BEST May/Fall

PERMITS None

RULES No beach camping in state parks or within sight of houses

CONTACT Nehalem Bay State Park, which manages Ecola and Oswald West parks, (503) 368-5943

SPECIAL ATTRACTIONS Magnificent coastal scenery; open year-round

PROBLEMS Crowded in spots; limited camping opportunities; tide concerns; early-season mud, washouts, and blowdowns

HOW TO GET THERE From downtown Seaside, the northern trailhead is reached by driving south on Edgewood Street (which becomes Sunset Boulevard) to the parking lot at road's end. Numerous access points allow you to shorten the trip in many places, but the recommended exit is the small gravel road on the south side of Neahkahnie Mountain reached off Highway 101 between mileposts 41 and 42.

INTRODUCTION This popular stretch of the Oregon Coast Trail packs a lot of scenic variety in a small area. From beaches and tidepools to dense forests and high viewpoints, this trip has it all. Add a dose of history and you have a great early- or late-season hike. May is best for flowers, but fall is also pleasant and has fewer people. The entire stretch can be done as a series of fairly easy dayhikes, but a backpacking trip is more satisfying for the connoisseur. The hike is equally attractive in either

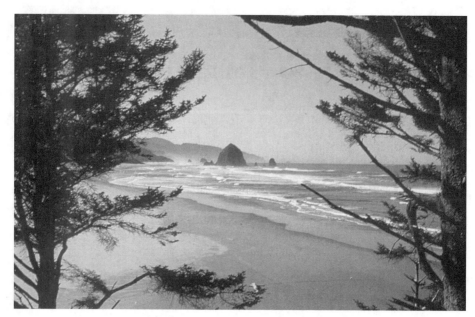

Looking south to Cannon Beach and Haystack Rock from Chapman Point

direction but is described here from north to south because that is the prevailing wind direction from late spring through summer.

DESCRIPTION You begin with a long climb through the second-growth forests of Ecola State Park. After 1.7 miles you reach the top of hulking Tillamook Head. A short side trail reaches the summit, which has rather disappointing views. The scenery soon improves considerably as the trail closely follows the edge of Tillamook Head's dramatic cliffs. Several places provide breaks in the trees with sweeping views of cliffs and ocean. Not necessarily the best but certainly the most interesting of these viewpoints is signed CLARK'S POINT OF VIEW. In 1806 Captain William Clark (of Lewis and Clark fame) stopped here with Sacagawea and other members of his party. In his journal Clark wrote that from here "I behold the grandest and most pleasing prospect which my eyes ever surveyed" (which is high praise considering all the wonders he had seen over the preceding two years).

The trail now drops 0.5 mile in a series of switchbacks to a four-way junction. Turn right to reach a backpacker's camping area and an old World War II concrete bunker. Nearby is a spectacular viewpoint several hundred feet above the pounding surf. Not far away is Tillamook Rock Lighthouse, which sits on a wind- and wave-swept offshore island. After dangerous and heroic construction efforts, this historic structure began operation in 1881 and continued its service until 1957, when it was abandoned.

Tip: A highly recommended book—fine reading material for this trip—is Tillamook Light by James Gibbs, a former lightkeeper on Tillamook Rock. His book masterfully mixes history with humorous anecdotes for a short but satisfying read.

Back at the four-way junction, turn south and steeply descend through a forest of ancient Sitka spruce trees.

Warning: This trail can be muddy and slippery when wet—almost anytime of year.

After 1.6 miles you reach the Indian Beach Picnic Area at the end of the Ecola State Park access road. Your trail continues on the opposite side of the road's turnaround loop. Cross Canyon Creek, then enjoy a very scenic 1.5-mile climb to the popular Ecola Point Picnic Area. There are several excellent viewpoints along the trail between these two picnic areas, particularly of the many offshore rocks and arches.

From the Ecola Point Picnic Area an excellent 0.2-mile side trip follows a paved trail to the breathtaking viewpoint at the tip of Ecola Point. The view must be shared with lots of tourists, but it's still worthwhile.

To continue your tour, relocate the Oregon Coast Trail near the picnic area's restroom and hike south. Cross a road leading to the park maintenance center, then top a small ridge where there is a superb viewpoint looking to the south. The trail drops a bit, then goes up and down for almost a mile before reaching the access path to Crescent Beach—well worth the side trip. The main trail goes straight from the junction and follows an often muddy route that features several nice viewpoints.

The trail joins a road shortly before the park entrance gate and follows it to another road, which drops into the quaint town of Cannon Beach. Here you have the option (unusual in the middle of a backpacking trip) to do some shopping, go to a nice restaurant, or spend the night in a luxury motel.

Tip: Plan to hike the next several miles of beach at low tide. This will allow you to explore the many interesting tidepools near famous Haystack Rock. In addition, the beach is more solid on the hard-packed wet sand of low tide, making hiking much easier, and three of the headlands require medium-to-low tide to get around.

Walk south along the popular beach and slowly leave civilization behind as you pass first Cannon Beach and Haystack Rock and then the smaller resort community of Tolovana Beach. Silver Point and, 0.7 mile

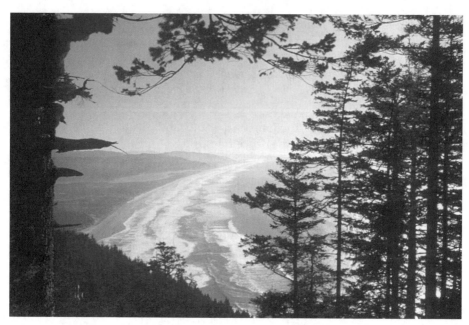
View south from Neahkahnie Mountain trail

later, Humbug Point can both be rounded at any tide other than high tide.

Warning: In winter, storms often erode the beach making it difficult to walk this section at anything but very low tide.

A moderately low tide, however, is needed to get around historic Hug Point, where the route is briefly an old roadbed. In the days before Highway 101 was built, the beach was the road between Cannon Beach and Arch Cape, and Hug Point represented a fairly significant obstacle. A narrow roadway was blasted into the rock here to allow vehicles to get around this point (one at a time) in between crashing waves. In addition to the historical interest, Hug Point features a scenic little waterfall, small caves, and picturesque sandstone cliffs. When the crowds aren't too bad, you can camp on the beach here (north of the point is quieter).

From Hug Point you continue south for 2 more miles of beach hiking to prominent Arch Cape and then turn inland to Highway 101. Cross the highway and walk 0.4 mile up Arch Cape Mill Road to Third Street. Turn right up a gravel road that becomes the Oregon Coast Trail and cross a suspension bridge over Arch Cape Creek. You climb forested switchbacks to a ridge saddle and then drop to another crossing of busy Highway 101.

The trail parallels the highway for a short distance, crosses an access road to Cove Beach, and then begins to enter wilder country. Your path climbs in long switchbacks through viewless second-growth forests to a broad ridge and then turns west through an area with lots of downed trees, testimony to the coast's sometimes vicious winter storms. As the trail drops down from the ridge, it passes near several dramatic viewpoints. First you'll be able to look north to Tillamook Head. After you round a ridge, there are views south to the cliffs of Cape Falcon. Wind-tortured snags add to the scenery—although this is no place to be when these trees are being tortured.

In a clearing choked with salal bushes, turn right to take the 0.2-mile spur trail to the dramatic viewpoint near the end of Cape Falcon. The view southeast up to massive Neahkahnie Mountain, the next scenic highlight, is particularly impressive. The main trail continues through woods to a confusing set of trails near tiny Short Sand Beach. Keep right at all junctions. The most important feature here for backpackers is Oswald West State Park's walk-in camping area on the west side of Highway 101 above the beach. There is a fee and you'll have to share the campground with people from the road, but it's still a pleasant place to spend the night.

To tackle the final obstacle, follow the scenic Coast Trail up three switchbacks and then along a view-packed route between Highway 101 on the left and the ocean's cliffs on the right. You cross the road at a large gravel parking area and begin the long climb of Neahkahnie Mountain. Views are intermittent but excellent on this heavily used forest trail. After 2 miles the trail breaks out into the large sloping meadows near the top of Neahkahnie Mountain.

Tip: Late May features a beautiful variety of wildflowers covering the slopes here.

Short side trails reach the summit's dual viewpoints. To complete your trip, traverse a wooded slope for 0.5 mile, cross a jeep road, and drop steeply to the gravel road on the peak's south flank.

POSSIBLE ITINERARY			
	Camp	Miles	Elevation Gain
Day 1	Tillamook Head Camp	4.5	1100
Day 2	Hug Point	10.4	400
Day 3	Oswald West Camp (with side trip out to Cape Falcon)	11.0	1200
Day 4	Out	5.5	1600

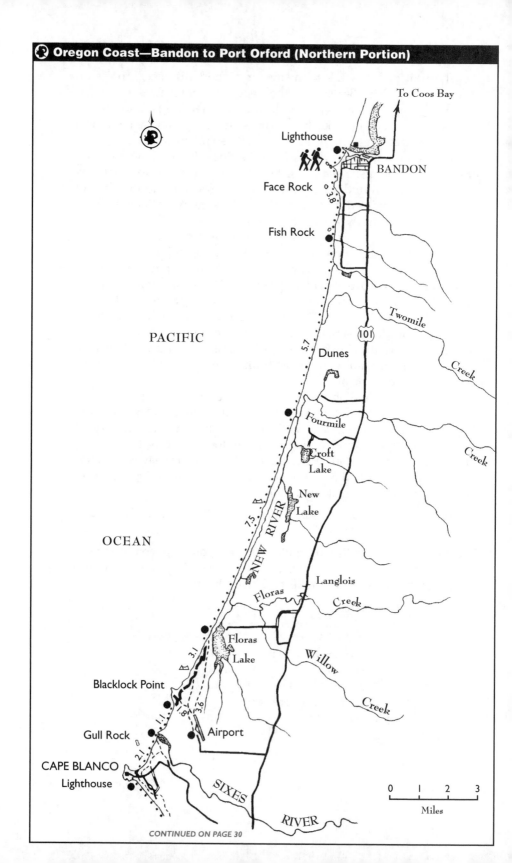

To Coos Bay

Lighthouse

BANDON

Face Rock

3.8

Fish Rock

PACIFIC

Twomile

Creek

101

Dunes

5.7

Fourmile

Creek

Croft
Lake

New
Lake

OCEAN

7.5

NEW RIVER

Langlois

Floras

Creek

Floras
Lake

Willow

3.1

Creek

Blacklock Point

.8

3.6

Gull Rock

1.1

Airport

CAPE BLANCO

2.1

Lighthouse

SIXES

RIVER

0   1   2   3

Miles

CONTINUED ON PAGE 30

2 Oregon Coast— Bandon to Port Orford

RATINGS (1–10)			MILES	ELEVATION GAIN	DAYS	SHUTTLE MILEAGE
Scenery	Solitude	Difficulty				
8	7	4	29	600	3-4	27

MAP None needed

USUALLY OPEN All year

BEST April to May/Fall

PERMITS None

RULES No beach camping in state parks or within sight of houses

CONTACT Oregon State Parks—South Coast Region, (541) 888-8867

SPECIAL ATTRACTIONS Coastal scenery; solitude; Cape Blanco Lighthouse; wildlife

PROBLEMS Tide concerns; frequent strong storms; hazardous stream crossings; parking concerns; beach closures to protect snowy plovers

HOW TO GET THERE To reach the hike's south end, leave Highway 101 just north of Port Orford on the marked road to Paradise Point. The road dead-ends at a picnic area and beach access. The north terminus is reached by following First Street through the charming town of Bandon and then Jetty Street to its end beside the south jetty of the Coquille River. Overnight parking is no longer allowed at the northern trailhead, and is not easy to find anywhere within more than a mile. Plan to be dropped off here, while leaving a car at the southern trailhead.

> *Tip: Regular bus service between the two cities allows you to do the trip without a car shuttle.*

INTRODUCTION For the most part, Highway 101 closely hugs the Oregon shoreline, rarely out of sight of the ocean. Between Bandon and Port Orford, however, the highway takes an inland course miles away from the beach. The result of this fortuitous decision by the road planners is

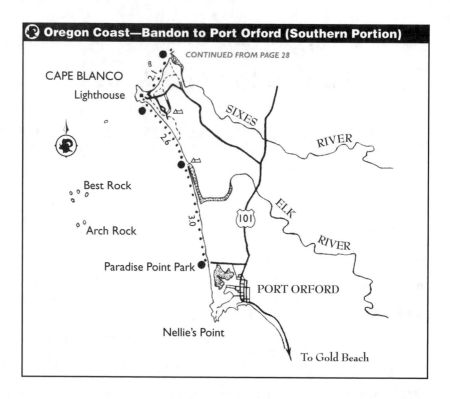

CONTINUED FROM PAGE 28

Oregon Coast—Bandon to Port Orford (Southern Portion)

CAPE BLANCO
Lighthouse

SIXES

RIVER

Best Rock

Arch Rock

101

ELK

Paradise Point Park

PORT ORFORD

RIVER

Nellie's Point

To Gold Beach

Oregon's quietest stretch of beaches and scenic headlands. This hike follows the state's only true wilderness beach, and deserves the attention of backpackers who love coastal scenery, wildlife, and wild surf.

> **Warning:** *Unless you are a strong hiker with experience in stream crossings, this trip is best done in late summer or fall. Crossing the Sixes and Elk rivers may be impossible early in the year.*

Since either direction is equally nice, the author's recommendation is to check the forecast and hike the direction with the wind at your back (usually north to south in summer and the reverse in winter—fall and spring are variable).

> **Note:** *To protect a nesting population of threatened snowy plovers, new regulations are in effect from March 15 to September 15. These require that for the first 11.5 miles south from the northern trailhead, hikers are required to walk on wet sand, have their dogs leashed at all times, and camping is strictly prohibited.*

DESCRIPTION If north to south is your chosen direction, the hike begins by your first admiring the cross-river view of the Coquille River

Lighthouse and then turns south along the beach. For the first few miles the route passes numerous offshore rocks and pinnacles. Table Rock is the largest one visible at present and, like the others, it supports a large population of nesting seabirds (numbers peak in May and June).

Tip: Hike this first 3 miles at low tide when the rocks are more accessible and picturesque. Avoid high tide, as the entire beach may be flooded with waves.

The sea stacks and pinnacles become more numerous and interesting as you approach Grave Point and Face Rock. A staircase connects up to a parking lot opposite Face Rock, so the beach here is crowded. The crowds thin considerably as you continue south another 1.9 miles to a scenic little cove called Devil's Kitchen. South of here, there is no easy road access for many miles so the beach is lonesome. To the east is a land of marshes and dunes that blooms profusely with yellow gorse in April. The beach is wide, smooth, and lovely all the way to Fourmile Creek.

The crossing of Fourmile Creek is easy late in the season but potentially hazardous after heavy winter or spring rains.

Tip: Bring a sturdy walking stick to act as a "third leg" for this and other stream crossings.

Not far inland, on the north side of the creek, is Lower Fourmile Creek Road. If the crossing is not feasible, you can use this road as an exit point.

The next 7 miles are basically more of the same—a wide, lovely, lonesome beach with nearby marshes and dunes. An added attraction is the New River—a slow-moving stream popular with both canoeists and wildlife. This "river" parallels the ocean for several miles, so you are actually walking along a sand spit.

Warning: Major winter storms sometimes break through this spit, making for difficult or impossible detours.

About 7 miles south of Fourmile Creek are the developments near large Floras Lake, over a low rise and a short distance inland.

Tip: If the winds are favorable, be sure to climb the foredune to take a look at this lake. Novice windsurfers practice here and are fun to watch.

Binoculars help. Two trails go inland from the southwest side of Floras Lake. The first starts very close to the lake's shore; the second (your route) begins further south after you pass a pond and reach a small cove.

South of Floras Lake the shoreline is characterized by bluffs and high cliffs. If the tide is moderate to low, take the time for a side trip down this beach. After 1.2 miles the beach ends near the base of a twisting waterfall. If there is a minus tide, it is possible to go around the base of Battleship Bow—as these cliffs at the north end of Blacklock Point are

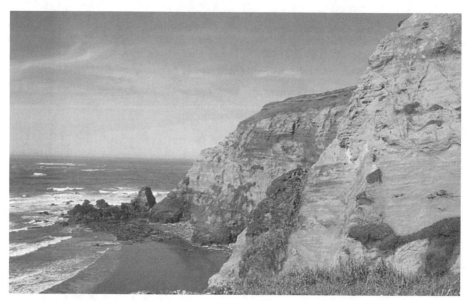

Cape Blanco

called—by scrambling over the beach's slippery boulders. The trail on the cliffs above, however, is easier and more attractive.

Taking the second inland trail from Floras Lake leads to a small creek with nearby meadows, trees, and a very attractive campsite. The poorly marked trail continues, mostly in forest, to a junction marked by a gray post. To the left is an exit to the Cape Blanco Airport. Your route turns right and alternates between forests and brush-covered meadows. Several short spur trails access a series of wonderful cliff-edge viewpoints. All of these are worth visiting, particularly the one featuring an excellent side view of the tall waterfall at Battleship Bow. One mile from the last junction is the next major junction. To the right is a not-to-be-missed 0.5-mile side trip to the meadowy headland of Blacklock Point. Offshore rocks and spring wildflowers add to the scene, which includes colorful sandstone soils and cliffs near the edge of the headland. Plan on spending at least an hour here exploring and just enjoying the view.

To continue your tour, drop down to the beach on the south side of Blacklock Point and travel another 1.3 miles to Sixes River. Recent changes in the river's course have made this crossing deep and potentially difficult. Unless you can find a convenient log jam (as often happens), plan on a tough crossing even in the low water of summer. Ask locals about conditions or scout it out from the nearby road in Cape Blanco State Park before you start your trip (see map).

Tip: Low tide is better because the river's water fans out across the beach, becoming a little shallower.

Leaving behind this obstacle, the next goal is obvious and enticing. Massive Cape Blanco juts out into the Pacific in open defiance of the strong waves and fierce winds that routinely pound this area. Picturesque Cape Blanco Lighthouse sends its flashing warning in all directions. The beach walk to this landmark is scenic and enjoyable.

Tip: Low tide makes the walking easier.

After 1.5 miles, just before the beach comes to an end, turn onto a trail that climbs the rolling meadow slopes to a road.

Tip: Don't miss the side trip west along this road to the Cape Blanco Lighthouse. Excellent guided tours are available most of the year.

From the lighthouse you have two options. The first is to go back to the road and follow a cliff-top trail through meadows and past viewpoints before dropping to the beach. This route passes near the park's pleasant car campground, a good choice for the night. The second option is more private and interesting: drop down the steep and trailless meadow slopes south of the lighthouse to reach a narrow beach. Walk this strip of sand and cobblestones past driftwood logs and offshore rocks.

Warning: This beach may be impassable at high tide and should not be attempted if there is a storm coming in. The wind and waves here are legendary.

After 2.6 miles the beach ends at Elk River, the trip's final major obstacle. In winter or early spring this stream is uncrossable and can be an adventure in any season after rain. Excellent camps can be made near the river. The final segment of beach stretches 3 miles south from Elk River to Paradise Point—the south terminus of your wonderfully wild coastal adventure.

POSSIBLE ITINERARY

	Camp	Miles	Elevation Gain
Day 1	BLM camp near New Lake	11.5	-
Day 2	Blacklock Point	7.6	200
Day 3	Elk River (with side trip to Blacklock Point)	7.8	400
Day 4	Out	3.0	-

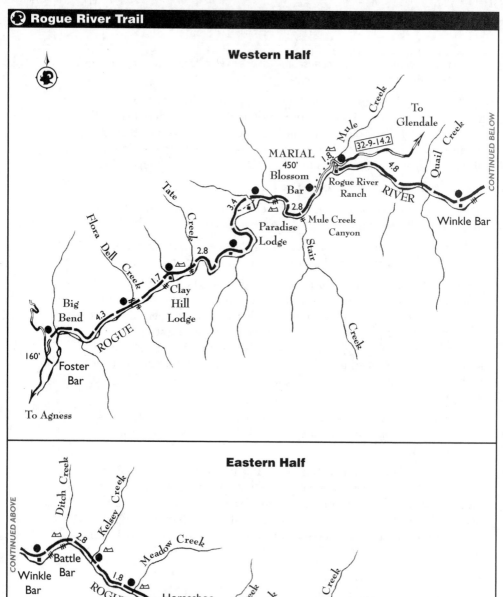

Western Half

MARIAL
450'
Blossom
Bar

32-9-14.2

To
Glendale

Mule Creek

Quail Creek

Rogue River
Ranch

RIVER

4.8

Winkle Bar

CONTINUED BELOW

Tate Creek

3.4

2.8

Mule Creek
Canyon

Paradise
Lodge

Stair

2.8

Creek

Flora Dell Creek

1.7

Clay
Hill
Lodge

Big
Bend

4.3

ROGUE

160'

Foster
Bar

To Agness

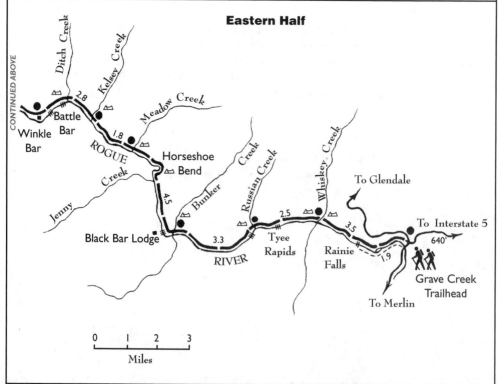

Eastern Half

Ditch Creek

Kelsey Creek

CONTINUED ABOVE

2.8

Meadow Creek

Battle
Bar

Winkle
Bar

1.8

ROGUE

Horseshoe
Bend

Creek

Jenny

Creek

Russian Creek

Whiskey Creek

To Glendale

4.5

Bunker

2.5

To Interstate 5

640'

Black Bar Lodge

3.3

Tyee
Rapids

Rainie
Falls

3.5

1.9

Grave Creek
Trailhead

RIVER

To Merlin

0   1   2   3
Miles

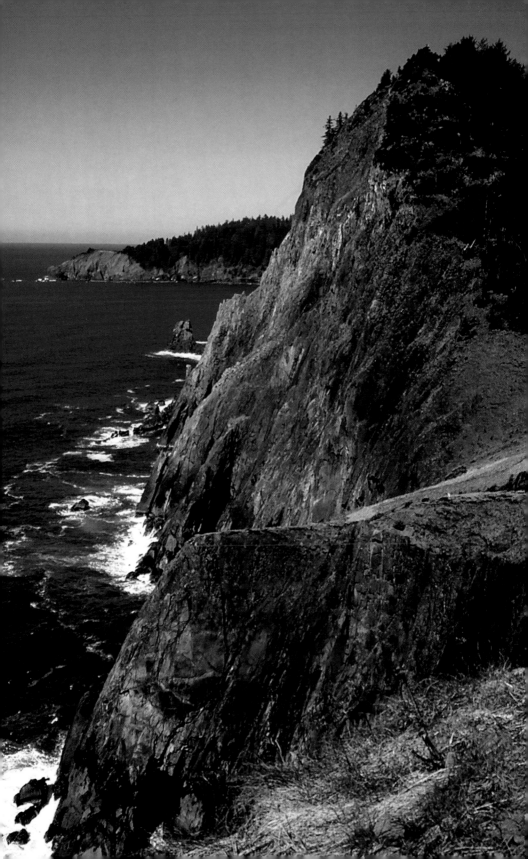

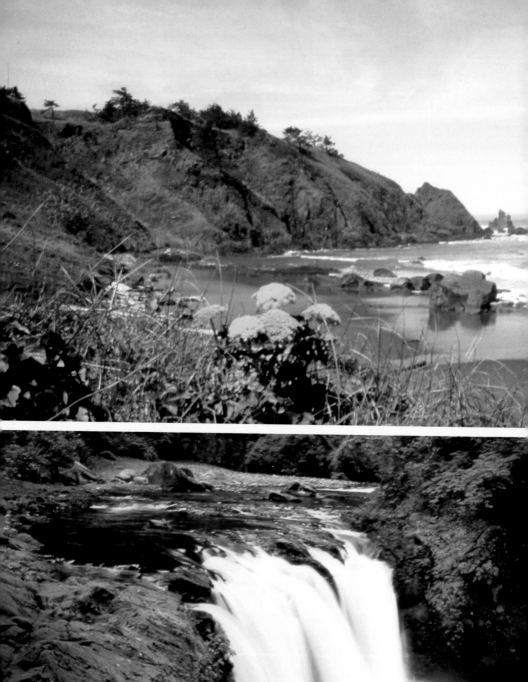
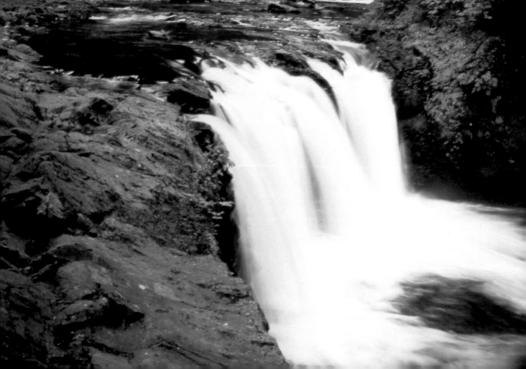

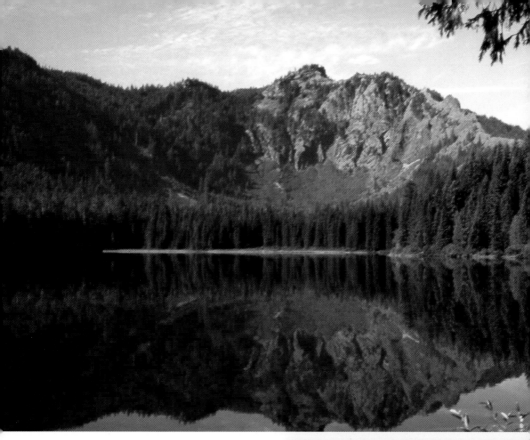

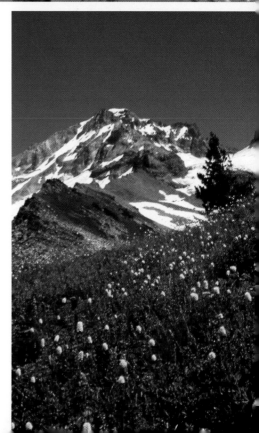

Previous page: Cliffs south of Cape Falcon (Trip 1).

Above left: Beach north of Cape Blanco (Trip 2).

Left: Lower Punch Bowl Falls, Eagle Creek, Columbia River Gorge (Trip 5).

Above: Mount Beachie over Elk Lake (Trip 6).

Right: Mount Hood from Yocum Ridge (Trip 7).

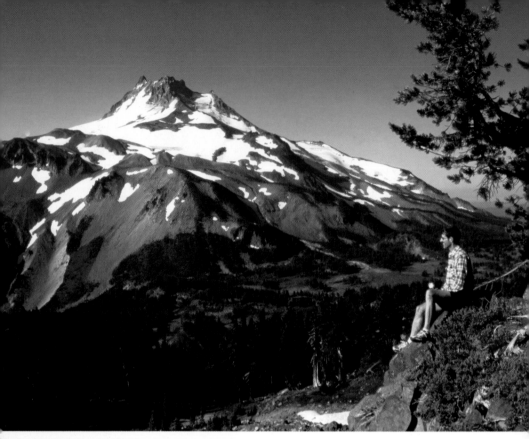

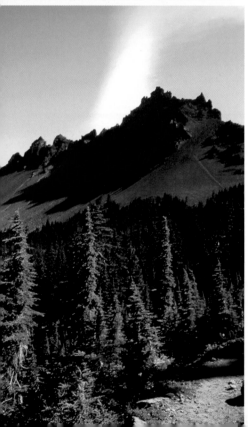

Above: *Mount Jefferson from Park Ridge (Trip 8).*

Left: *Three-Fingered Jack from the PCT (Trip 8).*

Right: *South Sister over lake in Green Lakes Basin (Trip 9).*

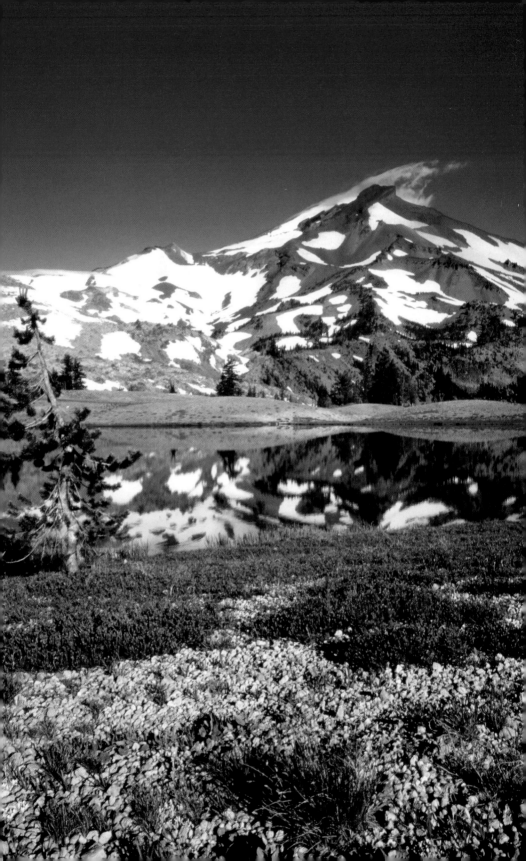

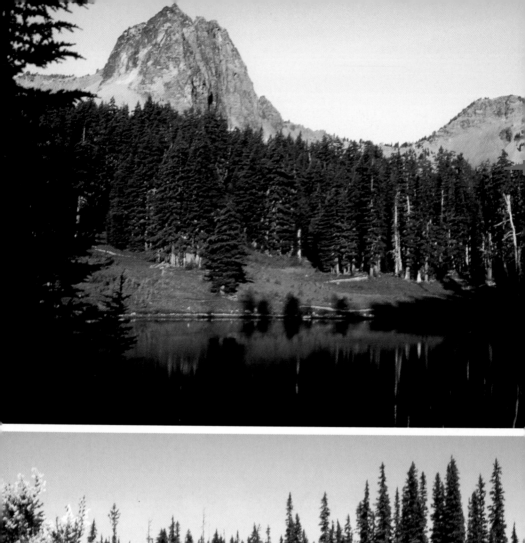
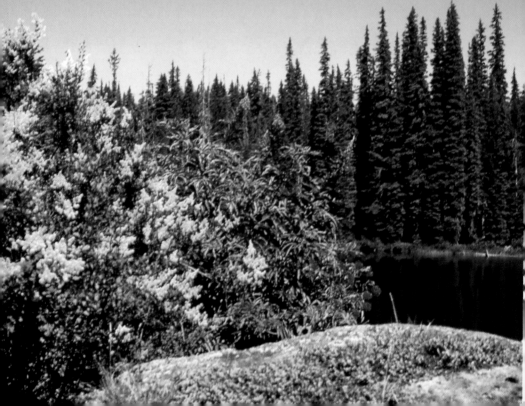

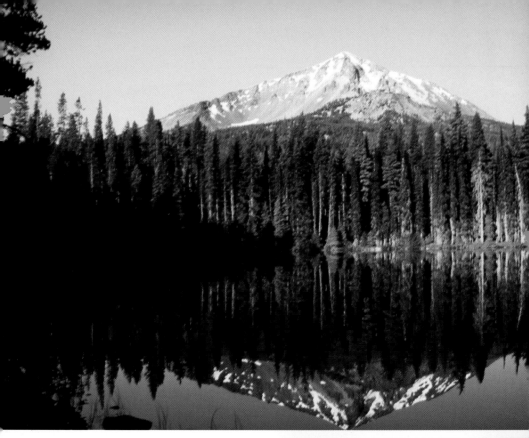

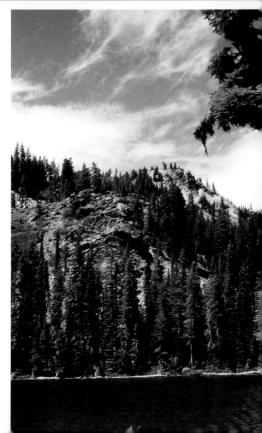

Above left: *The Husband over Husband Lake (Trip 10).*

Left: *Colorful display at Horse Lake, Three Sisters Wilderness (Trip 11).*

Above: *Mount McLoughlin over Squaw Lake, Sky Lakes Wilderness (Trip 14).*

Right: *Luther Mountain over Margurette Lake (Trip 14).*

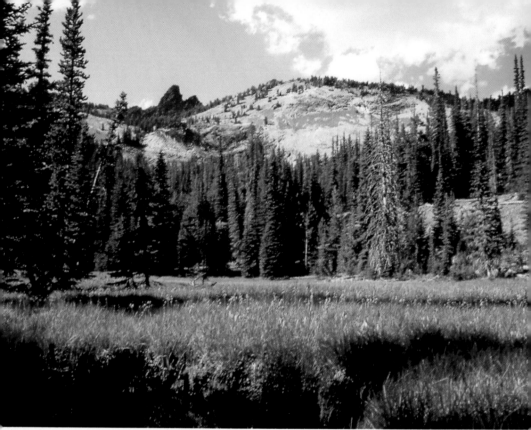

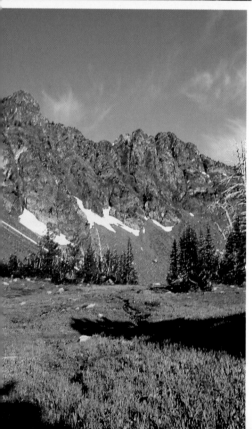

Above: Meadow below High Lake, Strawberry Mountain Wilderness (Trip 15).

Left: Ridge over Upper Twin Lake, Elkhorn Mountains (Trip 16).

Right: Wenaha River Canyon near Slick Ear Creek, Wenaha-Tucannon Wilderness (Trip 17).

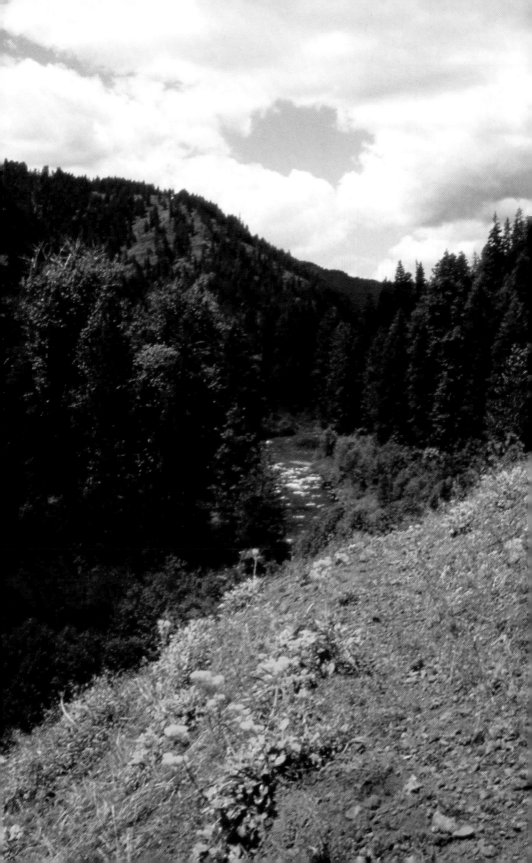

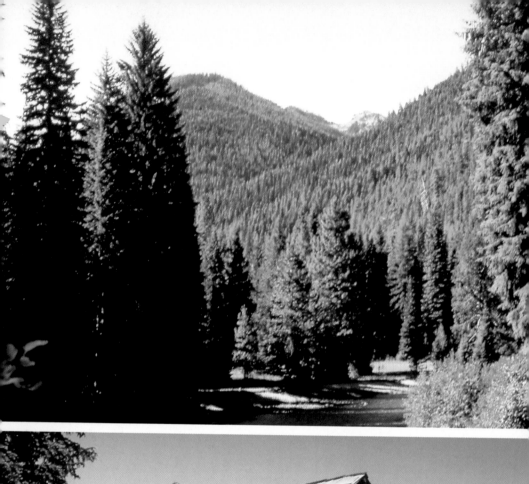
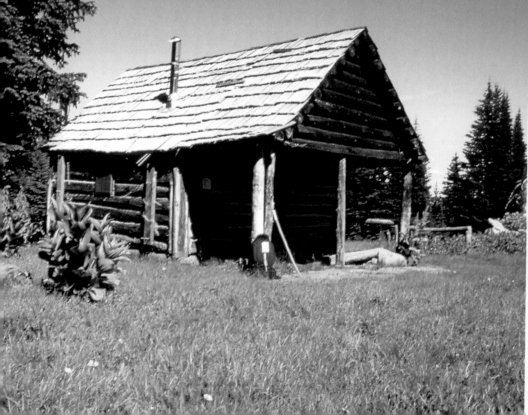

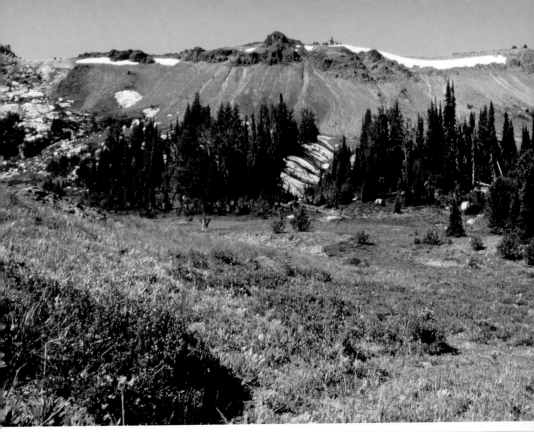

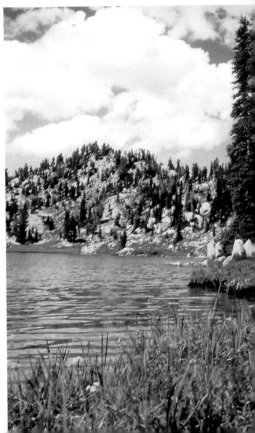

Above left: Minam River at Big Burn, Wallowa Mountains (Trip 18).

Left: Standley Cabin, Wallowa Mountains (Trip 19).

Above: Sturgill Basin, Washboard Ridge Trail, Wallowa Mountains (Trip 19).

Right: Northeast side of Swamp Lake, Wallowa Mountains (Trip 20).

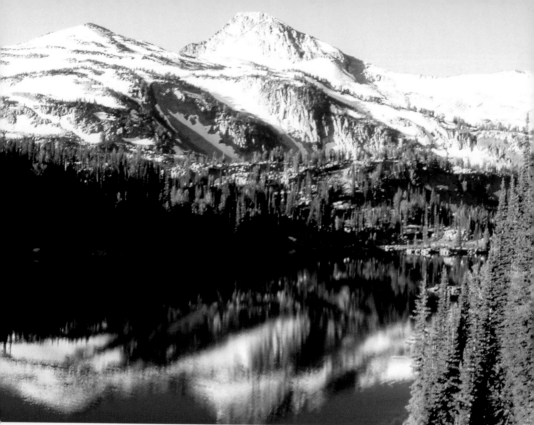

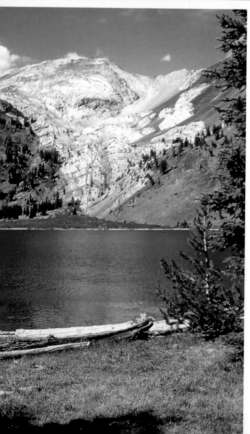

Above: Eagle Cap over Moccasin Lake, Wallowa Mountains (Trip 21).

Left: Peak 9775 over Ice Lake, Wallowa Mountains (Trip 21).

Right: Falls on South Fork Imnaha River, Wallowa Mountains (Trip 23).

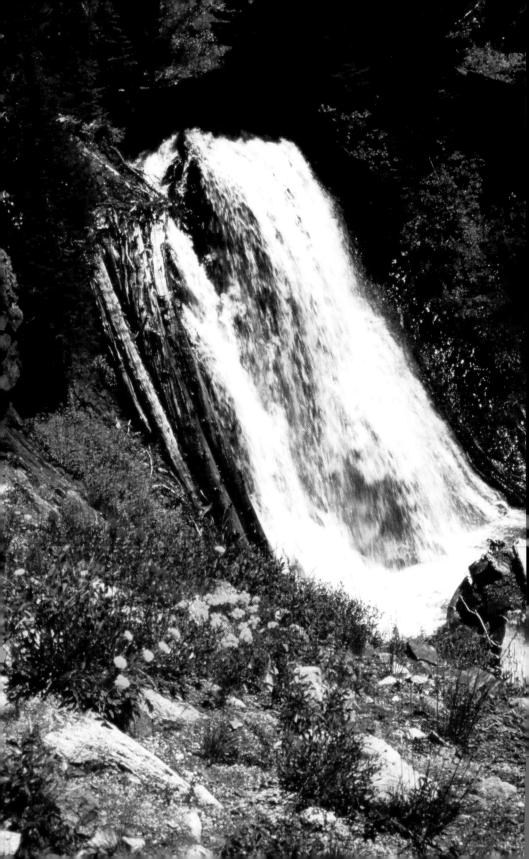

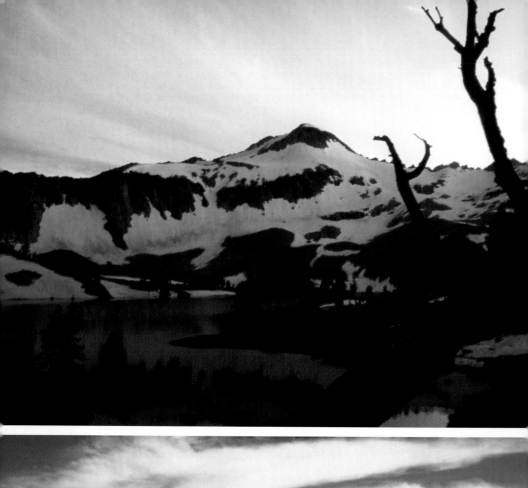
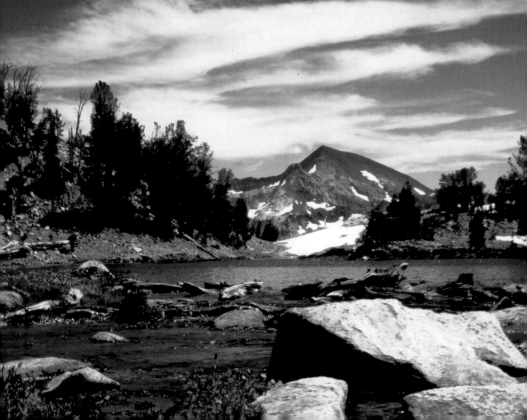

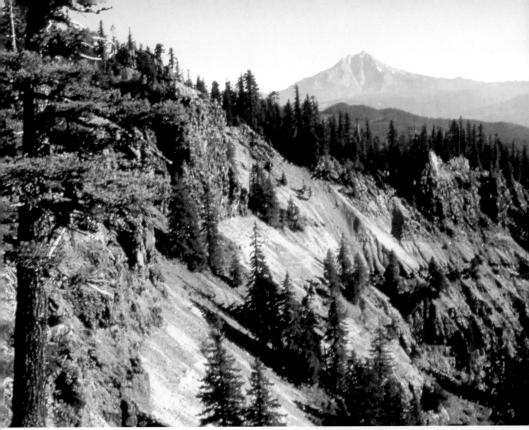

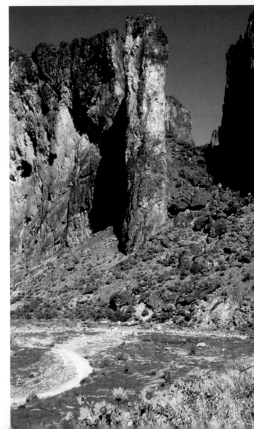

Above left: *Sunset at Glacier Lake, Wallowa Mountains (Trip 23).*

Left: *Sentinel Peak over outlet to Glacier Lake, Wallowa Mountains (Trip 23).*

Above: *Mount Jefferson over cliffs of Scar Mountain (Trip 33).*

Right: *In Three Fingers Gulch below Shadscale Flat (Trip 29).*

Following page: *Near the confluence of Whitehorse and Cottonwood creeks, Trout Creek Mountains (Trip 43).*

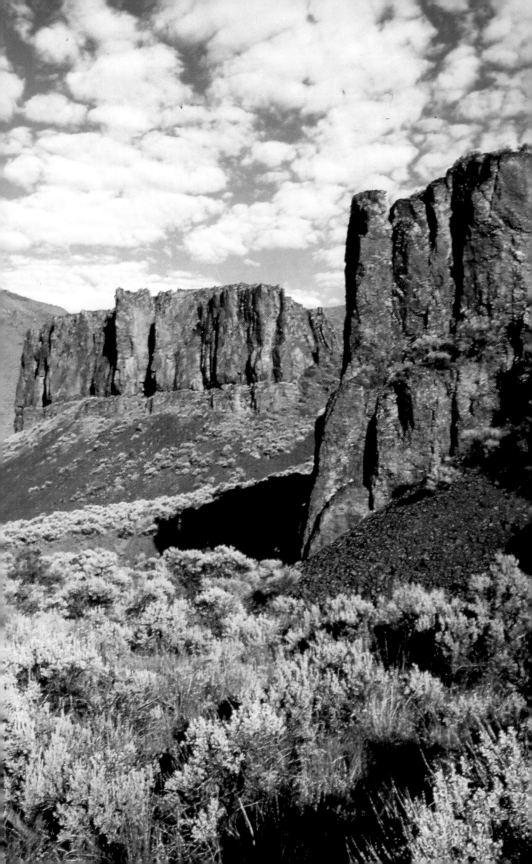

3 Rogue River Trail

RATINGS (1–10)			MILES	ELEVATION GAIN	DAYS	SHUTTLE MILEAGE
Scenery	Solitude	Difficulty				
10	5	4	40	3700	3–6	43

MAP USFS—*Wild Rogue Wilderness;* USGS—*Mount Reuben & Bunker Hill*

USUALLY OPEN All year (may be unhikeable in some winters)

BEST Late April to May/late October to early November

PERMITS None

RULES Fires prohibited within 400 feet of the river

CONTACT Grants Pass Office BLM, (541) 471-6500, and Gold Beach Ranger District, (541) 247-3600

SPECIAL ATTRACTIONS Outstanding river and canyon scenery; whitewater rafters to watch; waterfalls; wildlife; fall colors

PROBLEMS Profuse poison oak; rattlesnakes; ticks; summer heat; camp-raiding black bears

HOW TO GET THERE To reach the Grave Creek (upstream) Trailhead, drive 15 miles west from exit 76 on Interstate 5 to the Grave Creek bridge. Parking is available on the north shore at the signed trailhead and boat ramp. The lower (downstream) trailhead is reached by driving up the Rogue River Road for 31 miles from Gold Beach. Just after the bridge over the river, turn right and drive 4 miles to the Illahe Trailhead.

INTRODUCTION Southern Oregon's Rogue River has earned a special place in the hearts of whitewater rafters. The 40-mile float trip from Grave Creek to Illahe is one of the most popular in the country, and it's easy to understand why. This wild canyon provides continuously spectacular scenery, waterfalls, unusually abundant wildlife, and plenty of thrilling rapids. The Bureau of Land Management has a lottery system in place to regulate the number of people on the river. For backpackers there is an equally scenic way to see this roadless canyon. The Rogue River Trail has no crowds and requires no permits. The route parallels the north bank of the river for the entire distance. It is unquestionably one of Oregon's most exciting long backpacking trips.

Warnings: While the hike is undeniably outstanding, there are more than a few difficulties to keep in mind:

1) Poison oak is profuse along the entire length of the trail. It is sometimes difficult to avoid the stuff. Wear long pants and consider applying a preventive lotion before coming into contact with the plant's poisons.

2) Black bears have become used to raiding the camps of river rafters for food. The bruins are more of a problem here than anywhere else in the state. Hang all food (and anything else with an odor) at night and any time you leave your camp unattended.

3) Ticks and rattlesnakes are both fairly common. Take the usual precautions.

4) Avoid this trail in midsummer—the heat can be unbearable. Most of the trail is on sunny south-facing slopes, so bring a hat and plenty of sunscreen.

Probably the best way to see and enjoy the canyon is to hike upstream from Illahe to Grave Creek and then float down the river back to your car. The logistics of this plan, however, are rather complicated. For those who just want to hike the trail, an excellent option is to hike downstream and then use one of the shuttle services designed to take rafters back to their cars. Make arrangements with any of several commercial float-trip operators.

Tip: Many shuttle services will both drive you to the starting trailhead and pick you up at the end. This way you can leave your car at a safer location near the operator's business rather than the trailhead parking lot.

DESCRIPTION The HIKER ONLY trail starts with an easy stroll over mostly open slopes well above the river. Twisted oak trees provide frames for canyon photographs. You pass frothing Grave Creek Rapids, and then, at the 1.9-mile mark, reach Rainie Falls. Most rafters avoid running this dangerous section by using ropes to line their boats over a fish-diversion channel. A short side path leads to the base of this cascade. The main trail continues downstream, passes a nice sandy beach (a popular campsite for boaters), and then goes inland to the footbridge over Whiskey Creek. A short spur trail to the right leads to a historic cluster of mining machinery and cabins—well worth exploring. There are good camps near here for hikers setting a leisurely pace. The best camps are on a bench 0.4 mile west of Whiskey Creek.

To continue your tour, keep going west along the well-graded up-and-down trail generally staying on slopes 50–100 feet above the river. Pass Russian Creek's camps 2.5 miles from Whiskey Creek and then Slim Pickens Rapids in a narrow section of the canyon. After crossing Bunker Creek on a large bridge (good camp here), the trail begins to climb and enters a thicker forest of firs and maples on its way to Horseshoe Bend, where there are nice camps and a good view of this large loop in the river. More good camps tempt the hiker at Meadow Creek, but the ones just before the bridge over Kelsey Creek are even better. After passing Ditch Creek (a small camp here) and Battle Bar, the trail traverses an open grassy bench as it detours around pri-

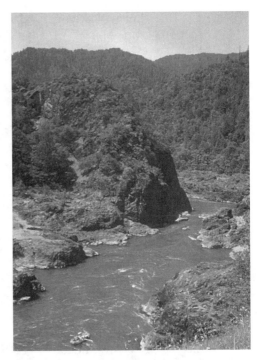

Rogue River and rafters below Paradise Bar

vate property at Winkle Bar. This is where Zane Grey, the famous western author, had a log fishing cabin. Unfortunately, there is no public access.

Near Quail Creek the trail returns to river level at a sandy beach.

Warning: *There are reports of arsenic in Quail Creek.*

The path now climbs back up the slope to detour around a slide and then passes through a 1970 burn area before reaching Rogue River Ranch, 23 miles from Grave Creek. This historic old home is now a museum and is listed on the National Register of Historic Places. It is accessible by car via the Marial Road, so don't expect to be lonesome.

Tip: *Be sure to schedule some time to tour the restored ranch and nearby exhibits.*

The Rogue River "trail" now follows roads for a short distance as it climbs to the Marial Road, crosses a bridge over Mule Creek near a car campground, and then follows the deteriorating dirt road to its end and the resumption of trail.

The lower canyon section from Marial to Illahe is even more dramatic and interesting than the upper canyon. In addition to the improved scenery, there are two trailside lodges that welcome hungry hikers.

Warning: Jet boats use this section of the river (at least as far up as Paradise Bar), so hikers can expect the tranquility to be interrupted occasionally by the roar of power boats.

You reach one of the major highlights of the lower river not long after the Marial trailhead. Beyond a short stretch through forests, you break out and follow a trail that has been blasted

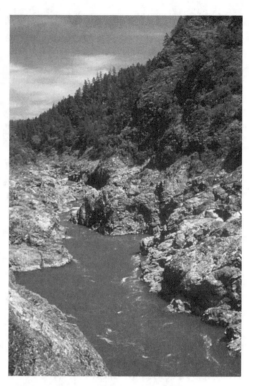

Rogue River at Mule Creek Canyon

into the cliffs above very narrow Mule Creek Canyon. At aptly named Inspiration Point there is a breathtaking view of this slot canyon. Adding even more to an already tremendous scene is Stair Creek Falls, dropping into the river across from you. After rounding this dramatic section, the trail reenters forests and then drops a bit to Blossom Bar.

Tip: Be sure to visit the river here as these rapids are one of the most challenging stretches for rafters. It makes for great fun watching them run the whitewater. There are nice camps near Blossom Bar Creek.

Continuing the trip, you soon reach Paradise Lodge, on a large meadowy flat above the river. Hikers can stop for lunch or even spend the night. For reservations, call *well* in advance at (888) 667-6483. Jet boats make scheduled stops here from May 1 to October 31. If you choose not to visit Paradise Lodge, the official trail detours around the meadow, staying in the perimeter forest.

Tip: Watch and listen for wild turkeys in this area.

After Paradise Lodge the trail follows the river around a prominent bend as the path cuts across a ridge called Devil's Backbone, which provides lots of good canyon views. The trail then crosses Brushy Bar—a forested flat that includes a ranger cabin, a creek, and several good campsites.

Warning: *Black bears are numerous in this area.*

From Brushy Bar the trail climbs to a historic high point signed CAPTAIN TICHENOR'S DEFEAT. In 1856 Rogue Indians overwhelmed a group of army soldiers under the captain's command by simply rolling rocks down the steep slopes onto the troops. Drop to Solitude Bar, another good place for viewing rafters, and then continue to the bridge over Tate Creek. Just below the bridge is a lovely waterfall. There are good camps here and 0.1 mile farther at Camp Tacoma. For more luxurious accommodations try Clay Hill Lodge about 0.5 mile ahead.

The trail crosses a long, sparsely forested section with plenty of river views on its way to Flora Dell Creek. Twenty-foot-high Flora Dell Falls has created an idyllic little fern-lined grotto and swimming hole just above the trail. Plan on spending extra time here cooling off and enjoying the scenery. The falls is a common dayhike goal for people coming upriver from the Illahe trailhead.

The final stretch of trail remains very scenic as it crosses open slopes with nice river views, especially of Big Bend. The trail climbs some 350 feet to make a detour around a landslide, but otherwise the hiking is easy. Impressive old-growth forests and several splashing side creeks add to the scenery. The last 0.5 mile is through an old apple orchard at the site of Billings Ranch. You may have to walk down the road a bit to reach the Foster Bar boat ramp, where commercial float-trip operators take out their rafts for the shuttle back to Grave Creek.

POSSIBLE ITINERARY			
	Camp	Miles	Elevation Gain
Day 1	Russian Creek	6.0	500
Day 2	Battle Bar/Ditch Creek	10.8	2000
Day 3	Blossom Bar	10.3	1700
Day 4	Out	12.9	900

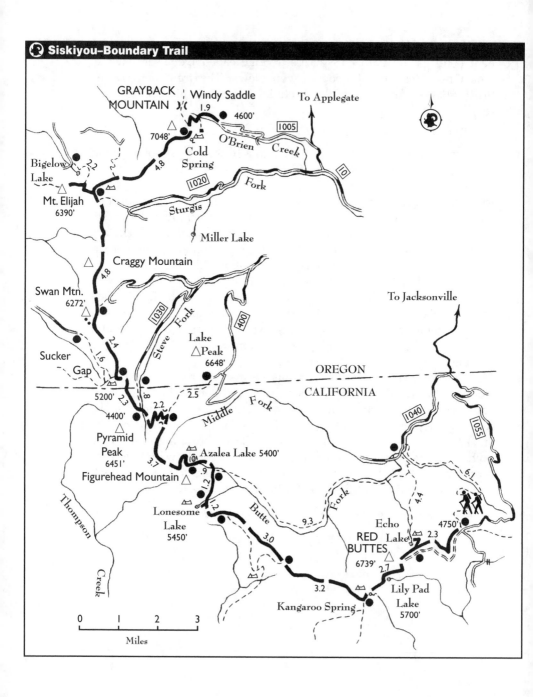

GRAYBACK MOUNTAIN

Windy Saddle
1.9
4600'

To Applegate

7048'

O'Brien Creek

1005

Cold Spring

10

Bigelow Lake
2.2

4.8

1020

Fork

Mt. Elijah
6390'

Sturgis

Miller Lake

Craggy Mountain

4.8

Swan Mtn.
6272'

1030

Steve Fork

To Jacksonville

Lake Peak
6648'

400

Sucker Gap

2.4

1.6

OREGON

5200'   2.3

.8

2.5

CALIFORNIA

4400'

2.2

Middle Fork

1040

1055

Pyramid Peak
6451'

3.7

Azalea Lake 5400'

Figurehead Mountain

.9

1.2

6.1

Fork

4.4

Lonesome Lake
5450'

1.2

Butte

9.3

Echo Lake

4750'

2.3

RED BUTTES
6739'

3.0

Thompson Creek

2.7

3.2

Lily Pad Lake
5700'

Kangaroo Spring

0   1   2   3

Miles

4 Siskiyou–Boundary Trail

RATINGS (1–10)			MILES	ELEVATION GAIN	DAYS	SHUTTLE MILEAGE
Scenery	Solitude	Difficulty				
8	7	5	37	8400	4	25
			(41)	(10,000)	(4–5)	

MAP USFS—*Red Buttes Wilderness* & USGS—*Grayback Mountain*

USUALLY OPEN Mid-June to October

BEST Late June to mid-July

PERMITS None

RULES Maximum group size of 8 people/12 stock; no camping within 100 feet of lakes; no camping or fires inside the Azalea Lake loop trail

CONTACT Siskyou Mountain Ranger District, (541) 899-3800

SPECIAL ATTRACTIONS Solitude; expansive views; wildlife; unusual geology and botany

PROBLEMS Black bears are common (hang all food and avoid areas with recent bear signs); cattle

HOW TO GET THERE To reach the east trailhead take Highway 238 southwest from Jacksonville for 8 miles to Ruch. Turn south and follow the paved road to Applegate Reservoir for 19 miles to a junction at the south end of the lake. Turn left and 1 mile later keep straight on gravel Road 1050 that goes up Elliott Creek. At a fork after 1 mile turn right onto Road 1055, which climbs 10 miles all the way to the Pacific Crest Trail crossing at Cook & Green Pass. To reach the O'Brien Creek Trailhead, the recommended exit point, return to the junction at the south end of Applegate Lake and turn west on Carberry Creek Road. Follow this good paved and gravel road for about 9 miles to a pass. Turn left on Road 1005 for 4 sometimes rocky miles to the hiker's trailhead at roadend.

INTRODUCTION The Siskiyou Mountains are unique. Nowhere else in the world is there a similar combination of converging climatic zones, merging geographic regions, and rare soils. The unusual east-west orientation of the range also helps to create a peculiar pattern of rainfall and ecologic zones. The result is one of the most diverse plant communities on the continent. There are both dry-zone plants and rainforest ferns; odd-looking endemic species live beside familiar favorites; alpine wildflowers grow next to sagebrush; and more different species of conifers live here than almost anywhere else on the planet (exceeded only by a few mountain ranges south of here).

But this area has more to offer than just unique flora. There is also a fascinating and highly scenic mix of rocks. Shining white marble intrusions mix with gray granite and green-black serpentinite, while in other places reddish-orange peridotite turns whole mountains its own special color. There are also small lakes and frequent views to enchant the visitor. Even the wildlife seems to agree about the attributes of these mountains, as they live here in an abundance unusual for the Pacific Northwest.

As the observant reader will note, a large part of the suggested route actually lies in California. The trip has been included in a book of Oregon backpacking trips for two reasons: first, because it really is too good to leave out; and second, from a practical standpoint, this truly is an *Oregon* hike. Road access is almost exclusively from the Oregon side, and the short car shuttle is almost entirely in that state. In addition, the nearest population center is Oregon's Rogue River Valley, where the Siskiyous are familiar landmarks. The hike is equally attractive in either direction but is described here from east to west as this involves less elevation gain.

DESCRIPTION   From Cook & Green Pass the Pacific Crest Trail, your route, heads southwest on a south-facing slope above a jeep road. South-facing slopes in these mountains tend to have only scattered trees but are choked with heavy brush. North-facing slopes have thicker forests with much less undergrowth. Excellent views extend toward the mountainous country to the south. At a pass covered with manzanita bushes is a junction. To the right is a steep but worthwhile 0.5-mile downhill side trip to Echo Lake.

The Pacific Crest Trail continues west, crosses the end of the jeep road, and contours around a ridge to Lily Pad Lake. The massive double summit of Red Buttes dominates the skyline. Grazing cattle and exposed terrain make this otherwise attractive pool unsuited for camping. Instead, continue hiking to the scenic basin holding Kangaroo Spring. Rare Brewer's weeping spruce is found near the PCT as you hike. The lush meadow at Kangaroo Spring is backed by the hulking form of reddish-colored Kangaroo Mountain and features a small pond and good camps.

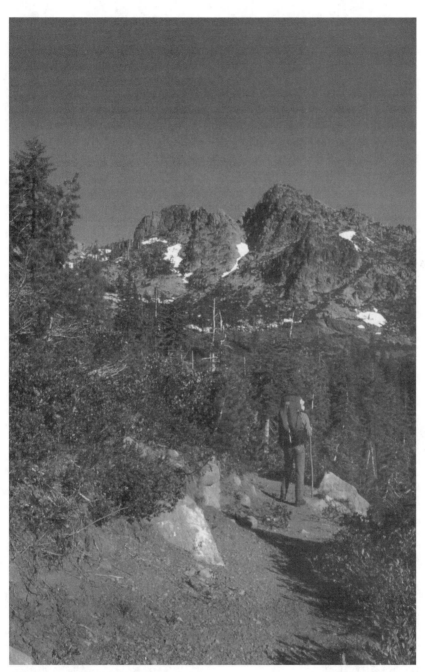

Pacific Crest Trail below Red Buttes

Tip: The next several trail miles have little or no water. Fill your bottles here.

As you climb away from Kangaroo Spring, the trail passes a particularly good example of white marble intermixed with the assorted other rocks of these mountains. At a ridgetop junction, the PCT heads south on its way to Devil's Peak and the Klamath River Canyon. Your route, however, turns right and contours across the south side of the main ridge for the next few miles. The trail passes beneath or beside ominously named places like Desolation Peak, Horsefly Spring, and Rattlesnake Mountain (none of which lives up to its name) before dropping to a saddle and a junction. The trail to the left goes down to Sugar Pine Camp. The more scenic alternative is to stay with the Boundary Trail as it closely follows the up-and-down ridgetop to Goff Butte. You pass on the south side of this peak and then climb over another high point in the ridge. Now drop to a small creek and look for the possibly unsigned junction with the trail to Lonesome Lake. The short side trip to this irregularly shaped pool is highly recommended due to its scenic setting, nice camps, and the reasonable chance of solitude.

To continue your tour, return to the main trail and follow the lake's outlet creek. The path goes up and down along the side of a mostly wooded ridge. You reach a marshy area with a nice view up to Figurehead Mountain and then drop to a junction in Cedar Basin. A fine collection of old-growth incense cedars accounts for the name of this place. The basin also has good camps, a wildflower meadow, and a pleasant stream.

Turn left at the junction in Cedar Basin and climb beside the creek to shallow but good-sized Azalea Lake. A trail circles this fairly popular lake, passing designated camping areas for both horses and hikers. Craggy Figurehead Mountain looms above the southern shore. From mid-June through July the air is filled with the sweet, pungent aroma of blooming mountain azalea—one of nature's most powerful and lovely perfumes. Of course, the colorful flowers also provide a treat for the eyes. There can be no question that Azalea Lake earns its name.

As you switchback out of this basin, the trail ascends through an open forest of lodgepole pine (unusual for these mountains) to a pass. The route then cuts across a rocky, view-packed slope to a saddle where knobcone pine and Brewer's spruce dominate. You loop north around the basin that holds Phantom Meadows and gradually descend a brushy sidehill with numerous views. Turn left at a junction and make a quick climb to a saddle with an excellent perspective of Pyramid Peak to the west before descending a series of long switchbacks into Steve Fork Canyon.

Just after crossing the creek is a junction. Turn left, make a switchback, and then begin a long, gradual, and usually dry climb northwest.

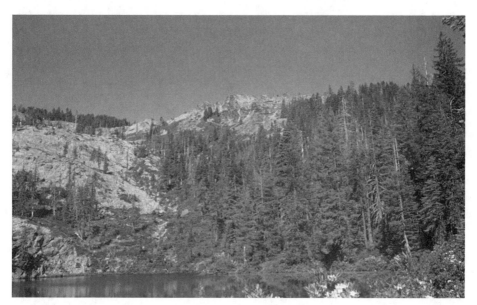

Lonesome Lake

Shortly after crossing a creekbed you'll pass into Oregon (the occasion apparently not worthy of a sign).

> *Tip:* At a sharp right turn about 2 miles from Steve Fork Creek look for a short, unsigned, unmaintained path that leads to a scenic lake in a cliff-walled little basin—well worth a visit.

The trail then climbs to a four-way junction at grassy Sucker Gap. The Boundary Trail turns to the right, but you first veer left for about 100 yards and then scramble down a steep trail to the lovely meadow beside Sucker Creek shelter. This meadow features a spring, lots of wildflowers, old-growth cedar trees, and welcome campsites. What may or may not be welcome are the black bears that seem to favor this basin. The author saw four bears here in one day—including one hanging around the shelter. Hang all food and camp away from the shelter, where bruins have become accustomed to finding bits of food. Deer are also common.

To continue your tour on the Boundary Trail, return to Sucker Gap and head north. The well-graded trail gradually climbs along the west side of a wooded ridge, eventually reaching a saddle with good views.

> *Tip:* For an outstanding side trip, climb cross-country 0.5 mile up a narrow brushy ridge to the top of Swan Mountain. The scramble is made easier by pieces of an old trail through the brush. At 6,272 feet Swan

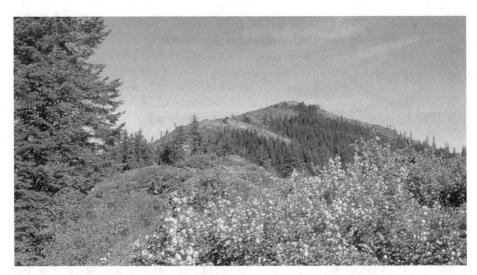

Swan Mountain from the Boundary Trail

Mountain provides an exceptional vantage point, particularly of the Oregon part of this range and the distant Cascade peaks to the east. To the north you can pick out Craggy Mountain, Mount Elijah, Lake Mountain, and Grayback Mountain—the string of scenic peaks that will occupy your attention for the next several miles.

From the saddle, follow the main trail north as it slowly descends the east side of a ridge. You pass an unmarked junction in a lush, sloping meadow appropriately called Green Valley and then climb back to another saddle. Now the trail loops around the west side of a hill and reaches a pass on the south side of aptly named Craggy Mountain.

Tip: *It is possible to scramble to the top of this peak, but the going is much steeper and more difficult than the route up Swan Mountain.*

Continuing to alternate between the east and west sides of the ridge, the trail leads around the east side of Craggy Mountain, passes below the remains of hard-to-find Denman Cabin, and then crosses a saddle back to the west. Shortly after the saddle, two springs just below the trail provide water, and as you continue north the path alternates between forest and open areas with nice views and lots of wildflowers.

Your trail now returns to the ridgecrest and crosses spacious Elkhorn Prairie. From this sloping meadow the trail descends to a junction in a forested saddle and then climbs briefly to a second junction. There is a nice sheltered campsite at this junction, with water from a spring 0.2 mile northeast along the Boundary Trail.

Tip: A worthwhile side trip goes left from here to the top of Mount Elijah—overlooking the Oregon Caves area. From partway along this side trail, you can also take a trail down to the wildflower meadow holding Bigelow Lake.

The main trail turns right at the junction, cuts across the south face of Lake Mountain, and then traces a tiring up-and-down course along the ridge to the northeast. Water is limited or nonexistent but there are some nice views.

At a forested saddle on the south side of hulking Grayback Mountain (the tallest peak along this ridge) the trail turns east and loops around the south side of this lofty summit. You round a ridge and pass just below the wooded area holding Cold Spring (good camps), from which an abandoned trail drops steeply to Krause Cabin. The main trail goes north across a large sloping meadow with several springs, wildflowers, and a sweeping look up at Grayback Mountain. Determined scramblers can reach the summit of this peak with its expected great views by making their way up steep meadows and then a rocky ridge. An easier side trip climbs the moderately steep trail to the north for 0.5 mile to the grassy pass called Windy Saddle, with exceptional views of its own.

To complete your tour, turn right at a junction with the O'Brien Creek Trail and descend a series of switchbacks to a junction just before the trail crosses O'Brien Creek.

Tip: Be sure to make a quick side trip to the right from here to visit a snow shelter and historic old Krause Cabin. The view up the sloping wildflower meadow from this cabin is excellent.

Back on the main trail, cross O'Brien Creek and complete the hike with a moderately steep descent through forest to the trailhead.

POSSIBLE ITINERARY

	Camp	Miles	Elevation Gain
Day 1	Kangaroo Spring (with side trip to Echo Lake)	5.6	1700
Day 2	Azalea Lake (with side trip to Lonesome Lake)	9.9	2400
Day 3	Sucker Gap	8.4	1800
Day 4	Bigelow Lake Junction (with side trips up Swan Mountain and Mount Elijah)	9.9	2700
Day 5	Out	6.7	1400

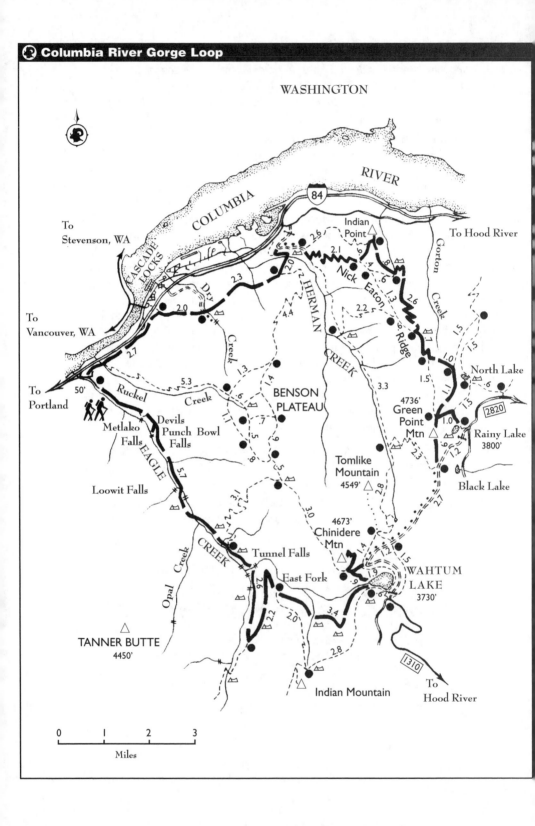

5 Columbia River Gorge Loop

RATINGS (1–10)			MILES	ELEVATION GAIN	DAYS	SHUTTLE MILEAGE
Scenery	Solitude	Difficulty				
6	5	6	39	6900	4–5	N/A
			(41)	(7800)	(4–5)	

MAP USFS—*Trails of the Columbia Gorge*

USUALLY OPEN Mid-May to November

BEST Late May to June/mid- to late October

PERMITS None

RULES Most trails closed to horses; camping allowed only at designated sites in lower Eagle Creek Canyon

CONTACT Columbia River Gorge National Scenic Area, (541) 308-1700

SPECIAL ATTRACTIONS Waterfalls; lush forests; very easy road access

PROBLEMS Crowded in spots; poison oak (at lower elevations)

HOW TO GET THERE Road access to the starting point is almost sinfully easy. Drive Interstate 84 east from Portland to Eagle Creek Exit #41. Turn right and park in the first lot on the left. The loop can be hiked in either direction but is more enjoyable going clockwise since this saves the spectacular Eagle Creek Canyon for the end.

Tip: The Eagle Creek Trailhead is very busy. On weekends arrive early to get a parking spot.

INTRODUCTION Close proximity to Portland and a wealth of easily accessible attractions ensure that dayhikers will always dominate the trails of the Columbia River Gorge. For those willing to invest more time in exploring the Gorge's wonders, however, a backpacking trip is ideal. This loop provides an excellent sampling of all the Gorge has to offer. There are deep forests, waterfalls, splashing creeks, high viewpoints, and cliffs. It includes busy trails beside major highways as well as rarely traveled paths in the remote backcountry. There is no better way to get to know and appreciate this special place.

DESCRIPTION Start by walking east 0.1 mile up the paved road toward the car campground. Turn left at a sign identifying gorge trail #400. The path passes around the north side of the campground before descending to an old concrete bridge over Ruckel Creek and a junction with the Ruckel Creek Trail. Continue straight, following the roadbed of the historic old highway for 0.8 mile through forests of Douglas-fir, bigleaf maple, and Pacific dogwood.

> *Tip:* The latter two species put on a fine show of color in late October and early November.

The route goes back to being a footpath but continues to stay close to Interstate 84. You wind through woods across from the Cascade Locks freeway exit and then meet a dirt road, where you turn left and go downhill to a signed junction with the Pacific Crest Trail. To the left is the Bridge of the Gods Trailhead (an alternate starting point).

Keep right, now following the PCT, as the trail climbs above some homes, makes a switchback, and then crosses under a set of power lines before reentering the forest. The surroundings rapidly take on a wilder character as you climb away from civilization. At the crossing of misnamed Dry Creek a jeep track comes up from the left.

> *Tip:* From the junction with this jeep road, a not-to-be-missed 0.2-mile side trip goes upstream to photogenic Dry Creek Falls.

The PCT heads east, passing two craggy rock pinnacles and a pair of lacy waterfalls. Turn left at a junction not far beyond the second waterfall and head downhill to a bridged crossing of Herman Creek. The trail then climbs gradually 0.4 mile to a junction. Turn right and quickly reach a jeep road, which you follow uphill to abandoned Herman Camp.

The Gorton Creek Trail begins at Herman Camp and provides an alternate way to continue your tour, but I prefer a steeper but more scenic route which continues straight on the old road for 0.2 mile, then turns left on the Nick Eaton Trail. This trail makes a long, moderately steep climb on numerous switchbacks. On the way up it crosses several large meadows that provide increasingly outstanding views and lots of wildflowers (blossoms peak about mid-May). Near the top of the ridge you reenter woods and reach a junction where you reunite with the Gorton Creek Trail. Turn left and follow this trail as it drops a bit to a junction where you turn right.

> *Tip:* After less than 100 feet look for an unmarked side trail to the left that drops steeply to the impressive rock pinnacle and viewpoint called Indian Point.

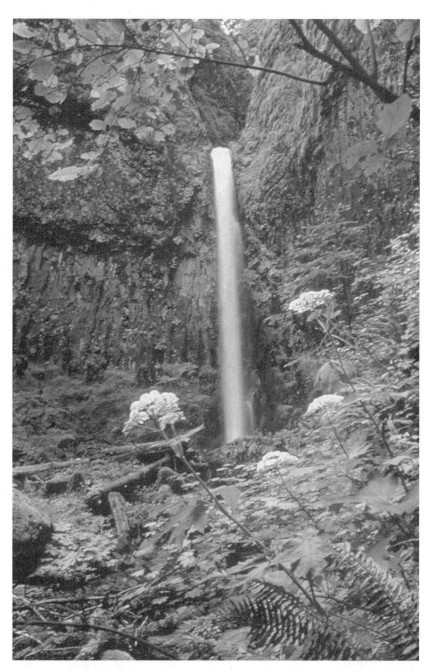

Dry Creek Falls

Back on the Gorton Creek Trail, the route then loses some elevation to woodsy Deadwood Camp, which is a good rest stop or campsite after all that climbing.

From the camp the trail makes a series of short switchbacks to a ridgecrest and then turns right to climb the spine of this ridge. Leave the crest and walk mostly down-hill across an area with numerous good views to the north and east. You cross a small creek and begin a fairly steep climb to a junction. Keep left along the east side of the ridge to a saddle holding Ridge Camp. Water is available along a path to the east.

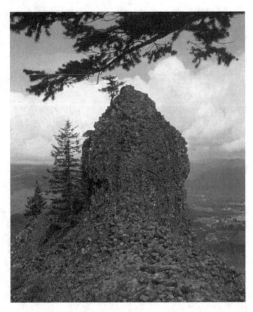

Indian Point

From Ridge Camp you switchback steeply uphill for 0.3 mile to a trail junction. The most direct route to continue your loop is to turn right and climb gradually through forests 1.5 miles to a junction below Green Point Mountain. A longer but more scenic alternative is to go left on Trail #412. This route climbs to a junction and then turns right, following the top of the cliffs above North Lake, where you will enjoy some excellent views to the east. Continue south to reach the previously mentioned junction north of Green Point Mountain.

> **Tip:** To visit scenic Rainy and North lakes, turn sharply left and drop to a trail junction. Turn right for Rainy Lake or left (straight) to reach more distant North Lake. Both have scenic settings and good campsites.

Back at the trail junction on the ridge, the path now climbs briefly to the summit of Green Point Mountain. Views are terrific from this high point. The distinctive mountain to the northeast is Mount Defiance, and the bald, sloping peak west across Herman Creek Canyon is Tomlike Mountain. The well-known Cascade snow peaks are also visible.

The trail continues south, dropping to a saddle where there is a junction with an old road coming up from the left. Keep straight, continuing on this "road." The route is often rocky, but views are frequent and excellent as the jeep road goes gradually up and down along the ridge. Just before the track turns sharply left, you leave the road and travel to the right a short distance to the Herman Creek Trail. At the next junction, this time with the Pacific Crest Trail, you have a choice. If you're tired or the weather is cloudy, turn left and make a long, gradual descent to popular Wahtum Lake. If your energy level and the weather allow, however, a better choice is to go right for 0.1 mile to another junction. Drop your pack and pick up your camera for an excellent side trip to the viewpoint atop Chinidere Mountain. To reach the summit, go straight on the PCT for 0.1 mile, turn right, and follow a moderately steep trail 0.7 mile to the top. Back at your pack, head left and switchback down past several possible campsites to the shores of large, tranquil Wahtum Lake.

Tip: Those interested in rare plants will want to keep an eye out for cutleaf bugbane, with its 5-foot-tall stalks holding plumes of small white flowers. This plant is found only here and at nearby Lost Lake. Excellent but often crowded camps are near the outlet of Wahtum Lake.

To complete your trip, follow the Eagle Creek Trail as it heads downhill beside Wahtum Lake's outlet stream. The trail turns away

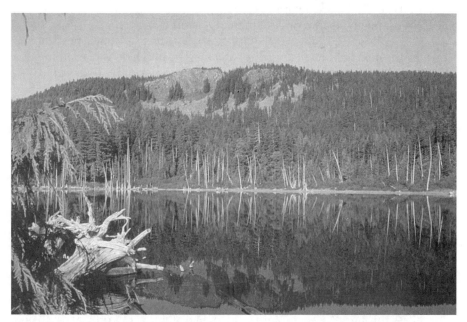

Green Point Mountain over Rainy Lake

from this creek but continues to lose elevation as it goes south to a side creek. There are more camps here—an alternate site if Wahtum Lake is too crowded for your tastes. The route maintains its consistent downhill grade as it crosses Indian Springs Creek and then continues to a junction with the Indian Springs Trail. Keep right (downhill) on the well-maintained Eagle Creek Trail to a sharp switchback on the ridgecrest with the appropriate name of Inspiration Point. The view from here of heavily forested Eagle Creek Canyon and rugged Tanner Ridge is superb.

The path turns sharply south, making a gradual descent along the side of a ridge. Cross a couple of small creeks with inviting campsites before you reach a junction with the little-used Eagle-Tanner Cutoff Trail.

Tip: *A nice, uncrowded creekside campsite is located about 0.5 mile up this trail.*

The main Eagle Creek Trail turns north, making the final descent to the banks of famous Eagle Creek. Despite the name, the author has yet to see any eagles here, but you might spot dippers (cute little gray birds that live in clear mountain streams). Something else you can't help but notice is the scenery. Cliffs draped with moss and ferns, lush forests, and a clear stream will be constant companions for the next several miles. Punctuating this lovely tapestry are a series of spectacular waterfalls. The falls are a variety of shapes and heights but are all beautiful. Bring plenty of film or card memory—you'll need it.

About 0.2 mile after the first waterfall, the trail comes near the top of the next falls, a tall, twisting cataract. The trail here is blasted into the basalt cliffs well above the chasm below. Cables provide handrails for those afraid of heights. Now you round a bend and immediately face towering Tunnel Falls.

Tip: *An extra-wide-angle lens is needed to photograph this massive falls.*

This falls gets its name because the trail has been dynamited through a tunnel in the basalt cliffs behind the falling water. In spring you can expect to get a bit of a shower as you round this exciting section. Tunnel Falls is the usual turnaround point for strong dayhikers coming up the Eagle Creek Trail. Expect to meet increasing numbers of people as you continue down the canyon. Try to hike this section on a weekday.

Hike through Blue Grouse Camp and then reach a junction with the Eagle-Benson Trail.

Tip: *Consider going up this little-used route for about 0.3 mile to some impressive viewpoints of the canyon.*

Pass through Wy'east Camp (which, like all the other official campsites in the canyon, is likely to be full of campers on weekends) and then cross the stream. Tenas Camp is on the left as you continue this joyously scenic canyon hike. A small waterfall is on Eagle Creek opposite this camp.

The great sights just keep on coming as you continue downstream. You recross the stream at aptly named High Bridge, where it's hard not to be impressed with the deep slot canyon below (despite the crowds of other admirers). Also impressive is the way the trail here has again been blasted into the side of sheer cliffs. Where the trail crosses an open slope there are some nice views of lacy Loowit Falls on a side stream across the creek.

Warning: Beware of poison oak here and throughout the lower canyon, especially in sunny areas.

The next highlight is an overlook that provides a nice perspective of short but very impressive Devil's Punch Bowl Falls. About 0.2 mile further a mandatory side trip drops to the left and then goes upstream to the pool at the base of Devil's Punch Bowl Falls, a world-famous photo spot. About 0.5 mile past Devil's Punch Bowl look for an unsigned side path that loops down to a fenced viewpoint of 100-foot tall Metlako Falls. The final 1.5 miles of trail generally stay well above the creek. The route, paved for its final 0.3 mile, ends at a busy parking area at the end of Eagle Creek Road. You must walk down the road about 0.4 mile to reach your car.

POSSIBLE ITINERARY

	Camp	Miles	Elevation Gain
Day 1	Herman Camp (with side trip to Dry Creek Falls)	9.4	1400
Day 2	Rainy Lake (with side trip to Indian Point)	10.1	4900
Day 3	Wahtum Lake (with side trip up Chinidere Mountain)	7.5	1400
Day 4	Out	13.6	100

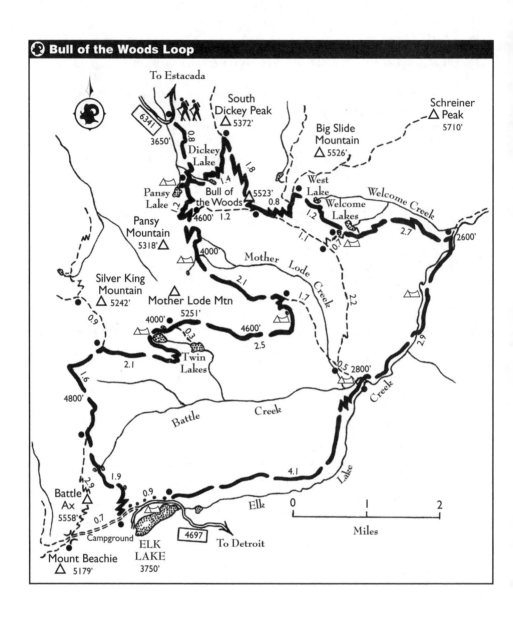

Bull of the Woods Loop

To Estacada

South
Dickey Peak
△ 5372'

Schreiner
△ Peak
5710'

Big Slide
Mountain
△ 5526'

634
3650'

0.8

Dickey
Lake

1.4

1.8

West
Lake

Welcome Creek

Pansy
Lake

1.2

Bull of
the Woods
4600' 1.2

△5523'
0.8

Welcome
Lakes

1.2

0.7

2.7

2600'

Pansy
Mountain
5318'△

4000'

Mother Lode Creek

1.1

2.2

Silver King
Mountain
△ 5242'

△
Mother Lode Mtn
5251'

2.1

1.7

0.9

4000'

0.3

4600'

2.5

Twin
Lakes

2.9

2.1

0.5 2800'

1.6

4800'

Battle   Creek

Creek

4.1

Lake

Creek

Battle
Ax
△
5558'

2.9

1.9

0.9

0
Elk

1

2

0.7

Campground

4697

To Detroit

Miles

Mount Beachie
△ 5179'

ELK
LAKE
3750'

6   Bull of the Woods Loop

RATINGS (1–10)			MILES	ELEVATION GAIN	DAYS	SHUTTLE MILEAGE
Scenery	Solitude	Difficulty				
6	7	6	29	6000	3–5	N/A

MAP   Green Trails—*Battle Ax* (#524)

USUALLY OPEN   Mid-June to October

BEST   Late August to mid-September

PERMIT   None (just sign the register at the trailhead)

RULES   Maximum group size of 12 people and/or stock

CONTACT   Clackamas River Ranger District, (503) 630-6861

SPECIAL ATTRACTIONS   Small, scenic lakes with good fishing; lovely forests

PROBLEMS   Irregular trail maintenance; mosquitoes in early summer

HOW TO GET THERE   From Estacada, drive 29.5 miles southeast on State Highway 224 then Forest Road 46 to a prominent junction with Forest Road 63. Turn right, following signs to Bagby Hot Springs, and proceed 3.7 miles to a fork. Go straight, still on Forest Road 63, drive another 2.9 miles, and then turn right on gravel Forest Road 6340. Stay on the main road at several minor intersections for 8 miles to a major fork, where you bear right, now on Forest Road 6341, and continue 3.6 miles to the Pansy Lake Trailhead. Parking is on the right; the trail is on the left.

INTRODUCTION   This trip explores a relatively little-known wilderness close to Portland, but a world away from that city's traffic and crowds. Although the wilderness has none of the eye-popping scenery found around major Cascades peaks like Mount Hood or the Three Sisters, it is still a lovely area, featuring numerous small lakes suitable for swimming or fishing, lots of huckleberries, and beautiful forests.

> *Note:* Unlike other trips in this book, the trails here are identified by number rather than name because almost all the signs at junctions in this wilderness only use the trail numbers.

DESCRIPTION Trail #551 goes south through an impressive lichen-draped forest of western hemlocks and Douglas firs that tower over the usual western Cascades understory of sword ferns, vine maples, Oregon grape, huckleberries, Pacific rhododendrons, and various forest wildflowers. The well-graded path steadily ascends for 0.8 mile, crossing several tiny creeks along the way, to a junction with Trail #549 and the start of the loop.

For the recommended counterclockwise circuit, go right on the main trail, which goes up and down for 0.2 mile to a poorly signed junction with the 120-yard spur trail to Pansy Lake. This side trip is well worth the minimal effort for the view of this shallow but scenic lake backed by the steep slopes and ridges radiating from Pansy Mountain.

The main trail bears left at the Pansy Lake junction and then makes two switchbacks up rocky slopes and through open forest for 1 mile to a junction atop a wooded ridge. Go straight and descend Trail #558, mostly in forest but with occasional glimpses through the trees of pointed Mount Jefferson to the southeast. A few irregularly spaced switchbacks help you descend to a low point at a campsite beside the trickling headwaters of Mother Lode Creek. Unfortunately, this creek is often dry by late summer and cannot be relied upon for water. Beyond this campsite, another 1.1 miles of up and down hiking leads to the next junction.

Bear right (uphill) on Trail #573 and gradually climb, still in forest, for 0.4 mile to a good and very scenic campsite on a small knoll above a pair of pretty, lily-pad-filled ponds. More climbing follows before you level off, finally losing about 500 feet to reach the Twin Lakes, 6.6 miles from the trailhead. An unsigned but obvious side trail goes sharply left to Lower Twin Lake. The upper lake, however, is more scenic and has better campsites, so stick with the main trail for 0.3 mile to the fine camps at that lake's west end. A rocky but delightful little swimming beach is nearby with easy access to the deep, clear water. It is usually comfortable enough for swimming from about late July to mid-September.

To exit the Twin Lakes Basin, follow the trail as it loops around the west end of Upper Twin Lake and then angles southeast, climbing a low ridge. Near the top of this ridge the trail winds its way back to the west and then continues gradually climbing. The forest here is dominated by higher-elevation species like mountain hemlock and western white pine, with frequent openings providing nice views of pyramid-shaped Battle Ax to the southwest. About 1.7 miles from Upper Twin Lake is a junction. Turn left (south) on Trail #544 and go up and down

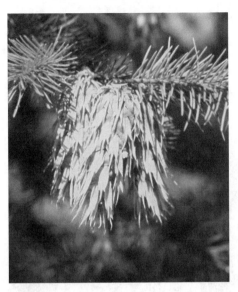

Young Douglas-fir cones

(mostly up) along an attractive ridge for 1.6 miles to a fork and a choice of trails.

The longer uphill trail switchbacks to the summit of Battle Ax where you will enjoy fine views up and down the Cascades and westward over the drainage of Battle Ax Creek. From there the trail switchbacks steeply downhill to the jeep road at Beachie Saddle, where you turn left and follow this rocky road downhill for 0.7 mile to a reunion with the lower trail.

If you prefer the easier and shorter trail, turn left at the fork north of Battle Ax, cross a rockslide, and then come to a small meadow with a fine view of Battle Ax. Just beyond here you pass two shallow ponds (no good campsites). The trail then crosses a brushy slope before passing another pond and descending four switchbacks to a junction with the jeep road coming down from Beachie Saddle, and a reunion with the upper trail.

Walk east on the jeep road, go straight at a junction with a better road coming in from a car campground on the right, and then walk through the forests north of large, tranquil, and very scenic Elk Lake. Near the western end of this lake, the road comes very close to the water and passes several excellent walk-in campsites that are well suited for backpackers.

Tip: The farther west you go, the better the views will be from your campsite across the lake to craggy Mount Beachie and towering Battle Ax.

Just before the road curves right to cross the lake's outlet, look for a sign identifying Elk Lake Creek Trail #559. Turn left onto this path, which despite its name goes nowhere near Elk Lake Creek for its first 4 miles. Instead, the trail contours for about 2 miles through relatively open old-growth forest and then gradually descends for 2.1 miles to a junction at a spacious camping area near the site of the old Battle Creek Shelter (now long gone).

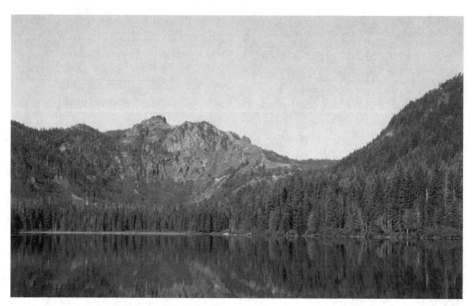

Mount Beachie over Elk Lake

Go straight at the junction here, still on Trail #559, and 0.1 mile later cross clear Battle Creek—an easy ford in early summer or a dry-footed rock hop by late summer. The up-and-down path then follows Elk Lake Creek through a lovely Douglas-fir and western-hemlock forest, with an understory featuring an unusual abundance of vine maples and Pacific yews. About 1.1 miles from Battle Creek is a bridgeless crossing of Elk Lake Creek. This ford is not dangerous, but you should expect your ankles and calves to get wet. The trail goes another 0.6 mile and then passes above a terrific (but chilly) swimming and fishing hole with deep clear water, lots of rising trout, and fine diving rocks. There is a small but very good campsite on the opposite side of the creek, reachable by scrambling down to the stream and then crossing the flow on a large log.

The trail now goes downstream another 0.9 mile, fords the creek a second time, and then climbs for 0.2 mile to a junction. Turn left on Trail #554 and begin a long, steady climb, always in forest and often through a jungle of tall Pacific rhododendron bushes. After climbing 1600 feet in 2.5 miles, you come to an unsigned junction with a 0.1-mile spur trail that goes downhill to the right to brush-lined Lower Welcome Lake. The main trail continues uphill another 0.2 mile to a good campsite and a junction just below small, lily-pad-filled Upper Welcome Lake.

Here you have another choice of trails. The slightly longer but more scenic recommended trail (#556) goes to the right through open forests and rocky areas where you will find a particular abundance of huckleberries—deliciously ripe in late August. The route also has pleasant views and passes above small and easy-to-miss West Lake. About 1.2 miles from Upper Welcome Lake is a ridgetop junction. Turn left on Trail #555, almost immediately pass a muddy pond, and soon come to another junction. Turn left again and then steeply ascend 18 short switchbacks to a junction with the optional trail from Upper Welcome Lake. Veer right, walk 0.3 mile, and reach another fork.

To finish your trip with the area's best viewpoint, bear right (slightly uphill) on Trail #554 and climb seven switchbacks in 0.7 mile to the boarded-up fire lookout atop Bull of the Woods. On a clear day this lofty grandstand provides views stretching from Mount Rainier to the Three Sisters as well as over the entire route of this trip.

From the summit of Bull of the Woods, go north (downhill) on Trail #550 that leaves just a few yards below the lookout building. This scenic trail descends intermittently along a ridge for 1.1 miles past rocky overlooks and through forest to a junction. Turn sharply left on Trail #549 and steeply descend for 0.9 mile to an unsigned junction with a 50-yard spur trail that goes to brushy Dickey Lake, which is set in a forested basin (no camps). The main trail goes right and continues downhill for 0.5 mile back to the junction with the Pansy Lake Trail and the close of the loop. Turn right and retrace your steps 0.8 mile to your car.

POSSIBLE ITINERARY			
	Camp	Miles	Elevation Gain
Day 1	Upper Twin Lake	6.9	1800
Day 2	East end of Elk Lake	6.2	900
Day 3	Upper Welcome Lake	9.7	2000
Day 4	Out	6.0	1300

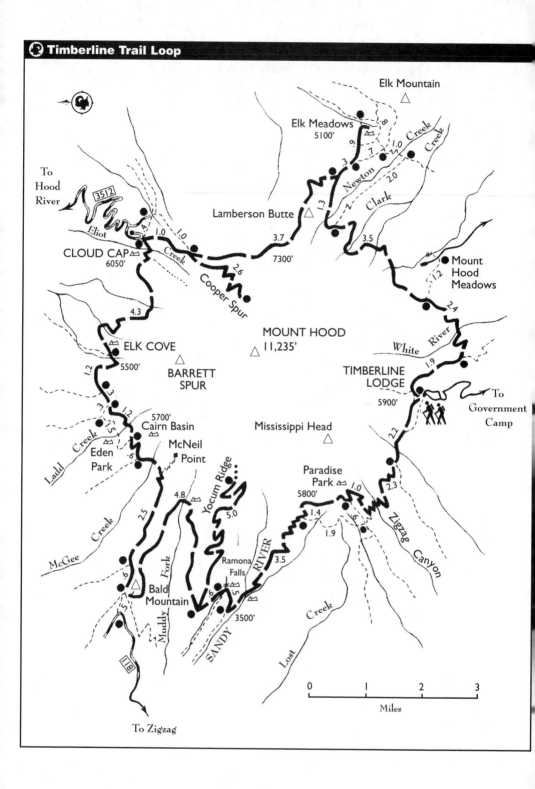

7 Timberline Trail Loop

RATINGS (1–10)			MILES	ELEVATION GAIN	DAYS	SHUTTLE MILEAGE
Scenery	Solitude	Difficulty				
10	2	7	41	8600	3–5	N/A
			(61)	(15,000)	(5–7)	

MAP   *Green Trails—Government Camp* (#461) & *Mount Hood* (#462)

USUALLY OPEN   Mid-July to October

BEST   Early to mid-August

PERMITS   Yes

RULES   Horses banned, except on the Pacific Crest Trail; no camping within 500 feet of Ramona Falls; no camping within 200 feet of lakes or streams; no camping or fires in meadows

CONTACT   Mount Hood Information Center, (503) 622-7674; Hood River Ranger District, (541) 352-6002

SPECIAL ATTRACTIONS   Great mountain scenery; wildflowers

PROBLEMS   Crowded; steep snowfields; unbridged glacial streams; proposed restrictions on permits and campsites

HOW TO GET THERE   Begin by driving to Timberline Lodge off Highway 26 above Government Camp.

> *Tip:* "Spacious" is hardly an adequate word to describe the acres of parking here. Don't forget to write down where you parked, or you might face hours of embarrassment trying to locate your vehicle when you return.

INTRODUCTION   The Timberline Trail circling Mount Hood is probably the most famous footpath in the state. Guidebooks describing the finest hiking trails in the nation often include this spectacular route, so Oregonians must share the trail with people from all over the country (and even international travelers). Even before the official trail was built by Civilian Conservation Corps workers in the 1930s, this round-the-mountain tour had many admirers—and justifiably so. The mountain views are stunning, wildflowers choke many of the meadows, and exceptional side trips abound. The enormous trail population is dominated by dayhikers,

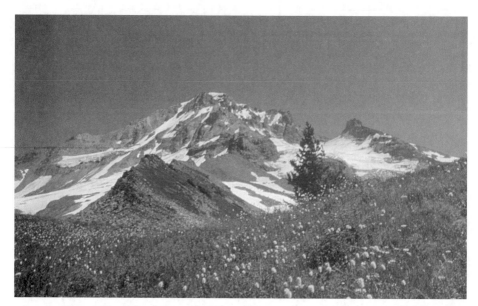

Mount Hood from Yocum Ridge

who have access to every corner of the mountain. The Forest Service has even considered restricting the numbers of hikers and campsites—an unfortunate but perhaps eventually necessary step. Because horses are banned from most of the route, the trails and meadows are still in good shape, despite the number of hikers.

It is traditional to start this hike at Timberline Lodge and travel clockwise. Almost all the backpackers who do the circuit choose this course, even though the trip is equally scenic in either direction, and can be begun at any of several trailheads. In a streak of contrariness, the author considered describing this hike counterclockwise and from a different starting point. The idea was dropped, however, for fear it would only lead to confusion.

DESCRIPTION From the back side of Timberline Lodge, follow a paved route signed TIMBERLINE TRAIL to a junction with the Pacific Crest Trail and turn left. The scenic path gradually loses elevation through flowery meadows and then crosses Little Zigzag Canyon. Keep right at the Hidden Lake Trail junction and continue losing elevation. The trail rounds a narrow ridge, where you will enjoy a fine view of Zigzag Canyon before dropping in long switchbacks to its bottom.

Warning: *The crossing has no bridge and may be wet.*

Climb back up the west side of this gorge to a junction. The horse route below Paradise Park goes left while the more scenic hiker's trail goes right and continues its long climb out of Zigzag Canyon.

In a sloping meadow covered with blossoms is a junction with the Paradise Park Trail. Keep right to reach the remains of an old trail shelter, near which there are many good but heavily used camps (please use a designated site). Although the camps are pleasant, trees and a small ridge block the view of Mount Hood from the shelter. You'll get better views as you continue hiking northwest on the up-and-down route for another 0.6 mile of flowers and unrestricted views before dropping back down to a reunion with the horse trail.

Brace your knees for a long series of downhill switchbacks as the trail descends 2,200 feet on its way into the Sandy River Canyon. Along the way are excellent views of the eroding cliffs of Slide Mountain.

Tip: Shortly before crossing the river is a nice, uncrowded camp beside Rushing Water Creek on the left.

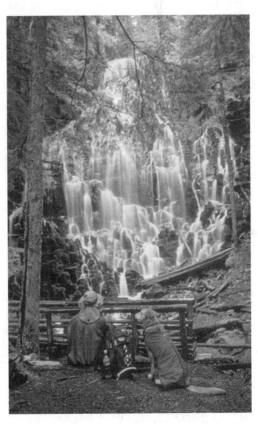

You cross the Sandy River and climb a bench on the far side to a junction with the popular Ramona Falls Trail coming in from the west. Make a sharp right turn and climb gradually 0.5 mile to Ramona Falls—a lovely curtain of water that cascades over a basalt cliff. Camps must be made at least 500 feet from the falls. A designated camping area is located to the south.

Warning: In recent years, trail damage on the northbound Pacific Crest Trail from Ramona Falls has caused periodic closures. Call ahead to see if you must detour to the west then north on other trails to rejoin the described route at Bald Mountain.

If the weather is good, the author *strongly* recommends you spend an extra day here with a long side trip up Yocum Ridge.

Ramona Falls

The trail leaves the PCT at a ridgecrest 0.6 mile northwest of Ramona Falls and makes a long but moderately graded climb through mostly viewless forests. Eventually the trail breaks out into wildflower meadows with a *terrific* view of Reid Glacier. By continuing on the trail for another mile and scrambling up a ridge you can also get up close and personal with the Sandy Glacier—*wow!*

Back on the main circuit, from the junction with the Yocum Ridge Trail the Pacific Crest Trail makes a long up-and-down traverse along the side of Yocum Ridge to a crossing of accurately named Muddy Fork Sandy River.

> **Warning:** *The ford of this multi-branched stream is a potentially cold, or even dangerous, adventure—especially on hot afternoons with lots of melting above.*

> **Tip:** *A clear stream a little north of the third branch of the Muddy Fork Sandy River has a good campsite and water that won't clog your filter.*

A long, mostly uphill segment takes the hiker up to Bald Mountain. The views back to Mount Hood from the steeply sloping wildflower meadows below Bald Mountain are outstanding. Now the trail loops back into the forest and soon reaches a major junction. The PCT heads off to the northwest, but our trail (Timberline Trail #600) turns to the right (east). You hike through a viewless forest, pass a trail junction, and then begin a steady climb up a ridge. Eventually the trail breaks out into ridgetop meadows featuring flowers and terrific views of Mount Hood. Make four switchbacks and encounter an unmarked but obvious side trail that climbs very steeply over loose rocks and roots to McNeil Point shelter (a tiring but worthwhile side trip).

Stick with the Timberline Trail and cross a basin with two small ponds.

> **Tip:** *Photographers will want to climb the small hill south of these ponds to a fine view of the top one-third of Mount Hood.*

The route climbs briefly over a ridge and then contours to the excellent camps in scenic Cairn Basin.

If you're camped at Cairn Basin and have time for some exploring, there are several possible options. You can make a lovely loop trip by dropping to the wildflower gardens of Eden Park, going east to Wy'east Basin, and returning to Cairn Basin via the Timberline Trail.

> **Warning:** *The loop requires two crossings of Ladd Creek, not always a lead-pipe cinch.*

Ambitious hikers should also consider making the trailless scramble up Barrett Spur. Leave the Timberline Trail near the junction with the Vista Ridge Trail and climb through meadows and over rocky slopes for about 1.5 miles to the summit viewpoint. The jumbled ice masses of Ladd and Coe glaciers are especially impressive.

The main Timberline Trail goes through continuously spectacular terrain on an up-and-down course to the east. Shortly before it drops down a sidehill ridge, an unmarked side trail goes right to tiny Dollar Lake, which has camps but only limited views. Just ahead is Elk Cove, one of the mountain's most impressive beauty spots. The Cove has a particularly striking view of the north face of Mount Hood and the white mass of Coe Glacier. Wildflowers choke the meadow and a clear brook provides water. Camps here must be made in the trees below the fragile meadow.

The magnificent circle route continues with a loss of elevation to the crossing of Coe Creek above two towering waterfalls (which you can hear but not see) and then climbs back to higher-elevation meadows. Look for frequent views north to Mount Adams and Mount Rainier. At the crossing of Compass Creek are views of two waterfalls— a short one near the trail and a taller one a bit further downstream.

Tip: From a ridge just west of Eliot Creek an unmarked path climbs the moraine beside Eliot Glacier to some great viewpoints above the ice.

You cross raging Eliot Creek on a plank bridge and then climb a bit to the road and campground at Cloud Cap.

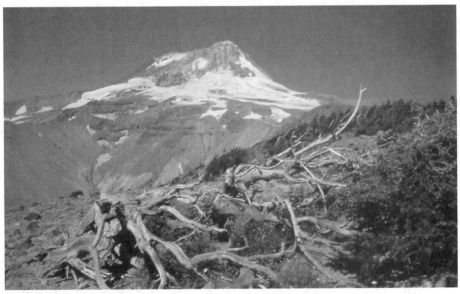

Mount Hood from Gnarl Ridge

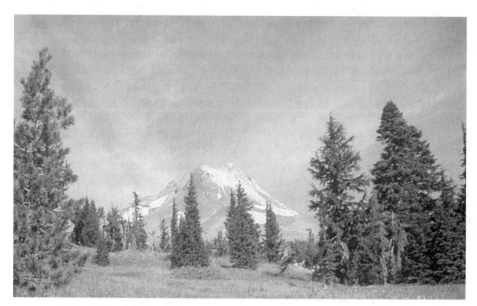

Mount Hood from above Mount Hood Meadows

Warning: *Severe flood damage closed the Timberline Trail at Eliot Creek in 2007 and required tough detours through 2010. Call the Hood River Ranger District for the latest conditions.*

The old inn near here is closed to the public, but this is still a popular trailhead with a campground to accommodate both car campers and backpackers. Tilly Jane Campground, 0.5 mile east, is another option for spending the night.

From Cloud Cap the Timberline Trail turns sharply southward, and skyward, as it climbs toward the highest part of the circuit. After 1 mile is a junction near a shelter.

Tip: *An outstanding side trip from here climbs in long switchbacks over talus slopes and snowfields to the viewpoint atop Cooper Spur. Before taking this side trip, keep in mind that it involves a round trip distance of 5.2 miles and an elevation gain of 1900 feet.*

The main trail goes south, climbing above timberline and crossing some steep snowfields.

Warning: *These snowfields are dangerously icy on cold mornings.*

Expect plenty of wind near the trail's high point on Gnarl Ridge before beginning a long descent into more friendly terrain. Above Lamberson Butte there are some great views across Newton Creek Canyon and up to Mount Hood. Massive Newton-Clark Glacier fills most of the mountain's east face.

The trail continues its long descent back into forests and meadows to a junction with the trail dropping to Elk Meadows. This large, popular meadow is well worth the 700-foot elevation loss and gain to make a visit. Highlights include an old shelter, excellent camps, marvelous views back up to Mount Hood, and a notorious population of gray jays that will happily eat from your hand (or steal your unguarded breakfast). To reduce damage here, the Forest Service asks that you camp in the trees around the perimeter of the meadow.

Back on the Timberline Trail, the route sidehills down to Newton Creek, which you can sometimes hop across, but a wet crossing is usually required. Pass a trail junction and then contour around a ridge before coming to Clark Creek, an easier crossing. The tour now passes through a surprisingly scenic area of wildflowers in the Mount Hood Meadows ski area. Ski areas are usually eyesores in summer, but this one isn't bad. There are even occasional views up to Mount Hood.

Leave the ski area and start a long 1,000-foot descent into the bouldery wasteland of the White River Valley. This stream has no bridge and is the last potentially difficult crossing. The trail crosses this unattractive valley and then climbs a long switchback up the far side back

POSSIBLE ITINERARY

	Camp	Miles	Elevation Gain
Day 1	Ramona Falls	10.9	1400
Day 2	Ramona Falls (with day trip up Yocum Ridge)	11.8	3400
Day 3	Cairn Basin	9.1	2900
Day 4	Cloud Cap Camp	7.0	1500
Day 5	Elk Meadows (with side trip up Cooper Spur)	11.3	3400
Day 6	Out	10.5	2400

into meadows. In a particularly nice meadow is a junction with the Pacific Crest Trail. Turn right and climb this often sandy route for 2 miles back to your car (*somewhere* in that huge parking lot).

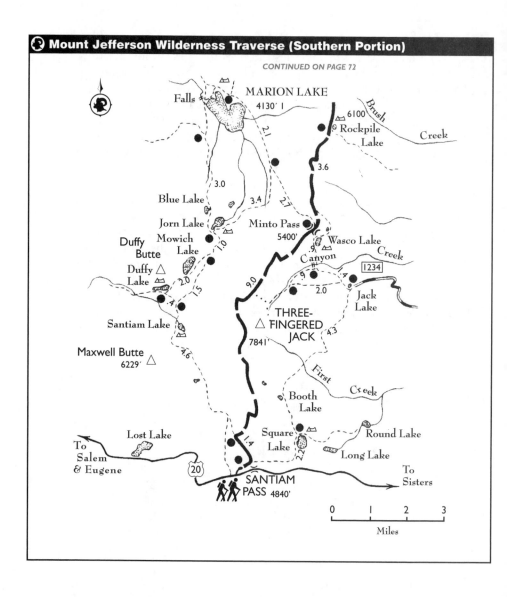

CONTINUED ON PAGE 72

MARION LAKE
4130' 1

Falls

Brush

6100
Rockpile
Lake

Creek

2.1

3.6

3.0

Blue Lake

3.4

2.7

Jorn Lake

Minto Pass
5400'

Wasco Lake

Duffy
Butte

Mowich
Lake

.9
Canyon

Creek

Duffy
Lake

1.0

.9

1234

2.0

9.0

2.0

Jack
Lake

Santiam Lake

1.5

.4

THREE-
FINGERED
JACK
7841'

4.3

Maxwell Butte
6229'

4.6

First

Creek

Booth
Lake

Lost Lake

Square
Lake

Round Lake

To
Salem
& Eugene

20

1.4

2.1

Long Lake

SANTIAM
PASS 4840'

To
Sisters

0   1   2   3

Miles

8 Mount Jefferson Wilderness Traverse

RATINGS (1–10)			MILES	ELEVATION GAIN	DAYS	SHUTTLE MILEAGE
Scenery	Solitude	Difficulty				
10	3	6	44	6400	4–6	76

MAP USFS—*Mount Jefferson Wilderness*

USUALLY OPEN Mid-July to October

BEST Late July to mid-August

PERMITS Yes

RULES No fires at Rockpile Lake or Jefferson Park; designated camp sites at Wasco Lake and lakes in Jefferson Park

CONTACT Detroit Ranger District, (503) 854-3366

SPECIAL ATTRACTIONS Views and mountain scenery; Jefferson Park—*wow!*

PROBLEMS Permits and access restrictions; long stretches without water; crowds; snowfields; crossing of Russell Creek; mosquitoes (especially in the Olallie Scenic Area) from mid-July to mid-August

HOW TO GET THERE Begin in the south from the well-marked Pacific Crest Trailhead off Highway 20 at Santiam Pass. The north trailhead is reached by taking Road 46 northeast from Detroit. Go over a pass after 16 miles, descend north another 7 miles, and then turn right (east) on one-lane, paved Road 4690. After 8 miles you turn right on gravel Road 4220 and continue another 6 miles to the trailhead at the north end of Olallie Lake.

INTRODUCTION The Pacific Crest Trail traces the entire mountainous backbone of Oregon. Along the way it visits most of the scenic highlights of the Cascade Range. Most hikers rank the section through the Mount Jefferson Wilderness as the best part of the PCT's route through Oregon, and it would be difficult to argue with them. The trail stays high for most of its length here, providing memorable vistas at nearly every turn. Continuing the trip north through the Olallie Scenic Area

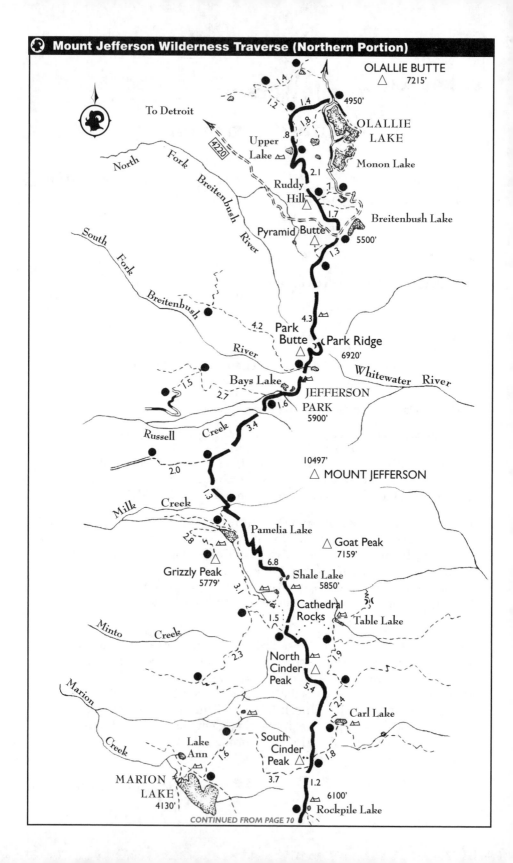

OLALLIE BUTTE
△ 7215'

To Detroit

North Fork Breitenbush River

South Fork

4220

Upper Lake ⌂

1.4
1.2
1.4
1.8
4950'
.8
2.1

OLALLIE LAKE

Monon Lake

Ruddy Hill △

7

1.7

Pyramid Butte △

Breitenbush Lake
5500'

1.3

South Fork Breitenbush River

4.2

4.3 ⌂

Park Butte △

Park Ridge
6920'

Whitewater River

1.5

Bays Lake

2.7

JEFFERSON PARK
5900'

1.6

Russell Creek

3.4

2.0

10497'
△ MOUNT JEFFERSON

Milk Creek

1.3

2.8

Grizzly Peak
5779'

△

Pamelia Lake

△ Goat Peak
7159'

6.8

3.1

Shale Lake
5850'

Cathedral Rocks

Table Lake

Minto Creek

1.5

2.3

North Cinder Peak △

1.9

5.4

2.4

Carl Lake

Marion Creek

Lake Ann ⌂

1.6

South Cinder Peak △∴

1.8

MARION LAKE
4130'

3.7

1.2

6100'
△

Rockpile Lake

CONTINUED FROM PAGE 70

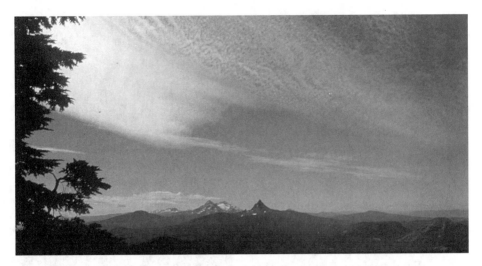

View south from the Pacific Crest Trail on the slopes of Three-Fingered Jack

adds even more lovely meadows and lakes. Hiking this additional section also eliminates the need to drive the *very* poor road to the Breitenbush Lake Trailhead.

DESCRIPTION   From the large southern trailhead parking lot, follow a short spur trail east to a junction with the PCT and turn left. Climb gradually through forest for 1.5 miles, passing a few stagnant ponds, to a junction with the Skyline Trail. Keep right and climb more steadily up the southern ridge of Three-Fingered Jack. The woods become more open and the scenery improves as you climb but the views of Three-Fingered Jack remain limited until you round a ridge and, rather suddenly, the trees break for a full frontal view of this craggy mountain. The trail crosses a talus slope and probably a few lingering snowfields, as it traverses the west and north faces of this peak.

> *Tip:* Shortly after a small pass north of the peak, look back for a final close-up view of Three-Fingered Jack's northeast cliffs.

The PCT then descends through forest and burn areas to a junction at Minto Pass. There are several designated camps at Wasco Lake a short distance southeast of the pass.

> *Tip:* A highly scenic alternate route to Wasco Lake drops steeply cross-country from the pass north of Three-Fingered Jack to spectacular Canyon Creek Meadows. These meadows have a terrific view of Three-Fingered Jack and support a riot of wildflowers in late July. Visit this popular spot on a weekday, and be extra careful not to trample the flowers.

To exit the meadows, hike the access trail to the northeast. Keep left at a fork (now paralleling Canyon Creek) and reach a small waterfall near a trail junction. Turn left (north) for another 0.7 mile to Wasco Lake.

Continuing north from Minto Pass on the PCT, slowly climb a heavily burned ridge and cross an open slope with fine views south back to jagged Three-Fingered Jack. Round a ridge and then reach the bowl holding Rockpile Lake. Fires are prohibited here. This small lake marks the beginning of an extended ridge walk featuring more great views than you can count. The only significant draw-back to this terrific stretch is a lack of water.

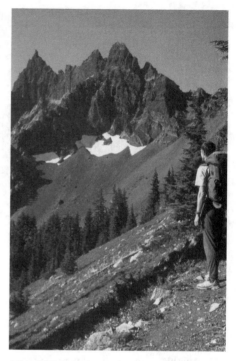

Three-Fingered Jack from the PCT

Only 1.4 miles north of Rockpile Lake is an open pass beside the reddish-colored summit of South Cinder Peak.

Tip: *Don't miss the easy scramble to the top of this cinder cone for an excellent view.*

The PCT continues its scenic route in and out of trees as it leads north toward the sharp spire of Mount Jefferson.

Tip: *At a small meadow shortly after rounding the west side of North Cinder Peak the trail passes an unseen shallow pond on the right, with water and a few camps. This is the only reliable trailside water between Rockpile and Shale lakes—a total distance of 8.8 miles.*

Not far beyond the pond is the first of several dramatic cliff-top viewpoints of Mount Jefferson and the diverse volcanic landscape below. This display of vulcanism includes cinder cones, lava flows, and a basalt-rimmed mesa called The Table. Only the Three Sisters area showcases a more interesting and scenic variety of the volcanic forces that shaped this landscape.

The trail drops a bit to the west and reaches a junction. Turn right (sticking with the PCT) and hike along the western side of the impressively rugged Cathedral Rocks. Next on the list of wonders is a partially forested plateau supporting several small lakes, of which only Shale and Mudhole lakes are near the trail.

Tip: These lakes are the jump-off point for excellent cross-country explorations to Goat Peak, to The Table, and, for the truly ambitious, up the long, steep south ridge of Mount Jefferson. Strong scramblers can get all the way to a point a little below the summit, where a dangerously exposed traverse stops those not equipped with climbing gear.

The Pacific Crest Trail gradually descends from the lovely high country on a series of long switchbacks to a junction with a trail coming up from popular Pamelia Lake. Nearby is a sweeping view up the steep canyon of Milk Creek to the top of Mount Jefferson. You cross Milk Creek and gradually climb to a junction with the little-used Woodpecker Ridge Trail. The trail passes a small, narrow lake with an unattractive campsite as it makes its way across the northwest side of Mount Jefferson.

Now you confront a potential problem—the crossing of Russell Creek. As with most glacial streams, this creek's volume increases significantly on hot summer afternoons, due to the melting of snow and glacial ice above. Try to cross in the morning, and expect a cold, possibly dangerous crossing—made worse by the brown glacial water obscuring possible footholds.

Not long after the crossing is a junction with the overly popular Whitewater Trail from the west. Keep right and follow the crowds to Jefferson Park, a nationally famous spot that should be seen by every Oregon outdoor lover. It is the perfect blend of alpine meadows, scattered trees, wildflowers, and lakes. Overlooking this scene is the snowy crown of Mount Jefferson. Camping near lakes is restricted to designated sites, and fires are prohibited.

Once you manage to drag yourself away from this paradise, the PCT climbs through more great scenery to the top of Park Ridge. Allow plenty of extra time to gaze in amazement here upon what many believe to be the best view in Oregon. The scene back down across the lovely expanse of Jefferson Park and sweeping up to the top of Mount Jefferson is impossible to describe.

To continue your trip, hike (or *slide*) down the huge semipermanent snowfield on the north side of Park Ridge. Relocate the trail and tour a scenic area of ponds, small trees, and heather meadows. Your route goes through a low pass and then turns northeast across a slope with views of prominent Pyramid Butte. Leave the wilderness and

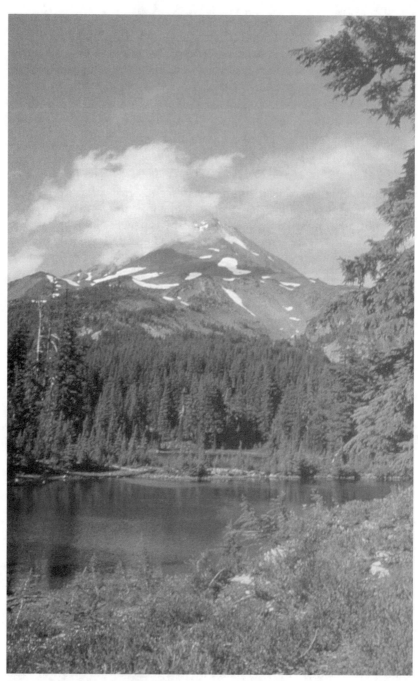

Mount Jefferson over Shale Lake

Backpacking Oregon

reach the trailhead near Breitenbush Lake on dirt Road 4220—an alternate stopping point for those with less time for hiking and a car they don't mind driving up this rough road.

The *recommended* exit point lies another 6 miles to the north at Olallie Lake. The route is continuously beautiful, if not as grandly scenic as the areas you've already seen. Go north around a shallow lake surrounded by meadows, wildflowers, and heather and then lose elevation past two quick junctions with trails from the east. Look for a short side path to the left up Ruddy Hill—well worth the 15-minute detour. The trail gradually descends to good camps beside shallow Upper Lake, backed by a scenic rockslide, and continues to Cigar Lake with its nearby ponds, meadows, and huckleberries. Continue north 0.5 mile to a four-way junction. Here you keep straight on the PCT for a final 1.4 scenic miles to the northern trailhead at Olallie Lake.

Warning: The lakes and ponds of the Olallie Scenic Area support a voracious population of mosquitoes. If you visit in July or early August come prepared with a headnet, insect repellent, and a willingness to do some swatting.

Note: The best option here for loop lovers is to follow the PCT to Milk Creek; take a day or two for a side trip to Jefferson Park; then return via the forested Oregon Skyline Trail past Pamelia Lake, Marion Lake, and Eight Lakes Basin.

POSSIBLE ITINERARY

	Camp	Miles	Elevation Gain
Day 1	Wasco Lake	10.6	1900
Day 2	Shale Lake	12.2	1500
Day 3	Jefferson Park	9.9	1800
Day 4	Upper Lake	9.5	1100
Day 5	Out	2.2	100

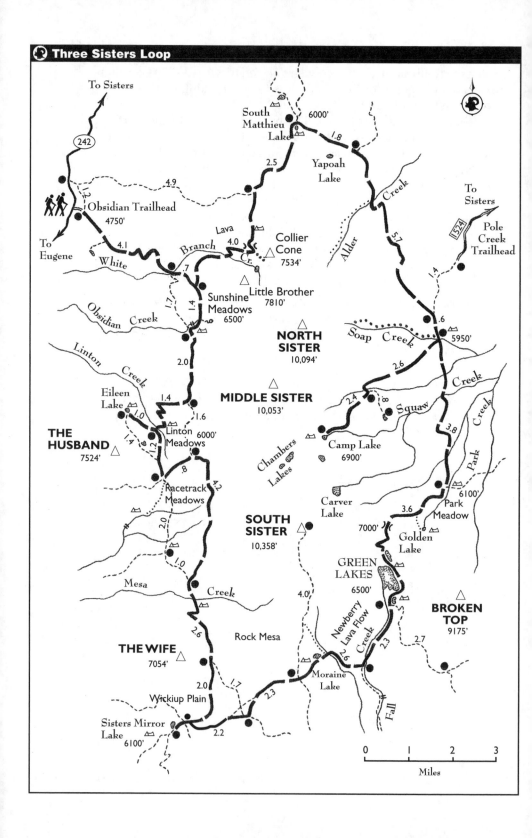

To Sisters

242

To Eugene

To Sisters

Obsidian Trailhead
4750'

1.2

4.1

.7

4.9

2.5

South
Matthieu
Lake

6000'

1.8

Yapoah
Lake

Alder

Creek

5.7

To
Sisters

524

Pole
Creek
Trailhead

1.4

Lava
Branch
Cr.

4.0

Collier
Cone
7534'

White

Obsidian   Creek

1.7   1.4

Sunshine
Meadows
6500'

Little Brother
7810'

NORTH
SISTER
10,094'

Soap   Creek

.6

5950'

Linton   Creek

2.0

Eileen
Lake

1.0

1.4

1.4

1.6

Linton
Meadows
6000'

THE
HUSBAND   7524'

1.2

.8

MIDDLE SISTER
10,053'

2.4

.8

Squaw

Creek

2.6

3.8

Park   Creek

Chambers
Lakes

Camp Lake
6900'

Racetrack
Meadows

2.0

4.2

Carver
Lake

1.0

SOUTH
SISTER
10,358'

3.6

7000'

Golden
Lake

6100'

Park
Meadow

Mesa   Creek

2.6

THE WIFE
7054'

2.0

1.7

Rock Mesa

4.0

Newberry Lava Flow Creek

GREEN
LAKES
6500'

2.3

2.6

BROKEN
TOP
9175'

2.7

Wickiup Plain

2.3

2.6

Moraine
Lake

Fall

Sisters Mirror
Lake
6100'

2.2

0   1   2   3

Miles

9 Three Sisters Loop

RATINGS (1–10)			MILES	ELEVATION GAIN	DAYS	SHUTTLE MILEAGE
Scenery	Solitude	Difficulty				
10	2	6	55	8200	5–6	N/A
			(75)	(10,600)	(6–10)	

MAP Geographics—*Three Sisters Wilderness*

USUALLY OPEN Mid-July to October

BEST August

PERMITS Yes

RULES No fires at Chambers, Eileen, Golden, Green, Moraine, or Sisters Mirror lakes, or Park Meadow; designated camps at Green, Moraine, and Matthieu lakes; limited-access permit required for the Obsidian area

CONTACT Sisters Ranger District, (541) 549-7700, and McKenzie River Ranger District, (541) 822-3381

SPECIAL ATTRACTIONS Terrific mountain scenery; interesting volcanic geology

PROBLEMS Crowds; permit and access restrictions

HOW TO GET THERE Follow Highway 242 (the McKenzie Pass Road) west from Sisters or east from McKenzie Bridge to the well-marked Obsidian Trailhead, just 0.5 mile south of the Scott Lake turnoff.

> **Warning:** This is a popular trailhead leading to an overly populated area (the Sunshine Meadows), so don't expect to be lonesome. You'll also need a limited entry permit (available from the McKenzie River Ranger District).

INTRODUCTION One of Oregon's greatest long backpacking trips, this route completely circles the Three Sisters, providing ever-changing views of these beautiful siblings. It also visits lesser-known family members (Little Brother, The Husband, and The Wife)—and craggy Broken Top, an apparent outcast, without family ties. The basic loop is unsurpassed, and countless side trips visit even more lakes, high meadows, and viewpoints. A hiker could spend weeks here and never tire of the scenery or run out of places to explore. So get your permit and savor this area.

Volcanic features dominate the landscape. In addition to rugged lava flows, cinder cones, and glasslike obsidian, you'll also see pumice meadows. Formed when enormous quantities of pumice bury an area, these meadows have sparse vegetation and no surface water. Examples of this geologic oddity include Racetrack Meadows and Wickiup Plain.

DESCRIPTION   The Obsidian Trail starts by climbing gradually through viewless forests. After 3.5 sometimes dusty miles the trail crosses a lava flow for 0.6 mile and comes to White Branch Creek. This stream often runs dry as the water percolates into the porous volcanic soils. On the far side is a junction. To the right is the most direct route to pick up the main loop trail, but any hiker not suffering from "destinationitis" should turn left. Although this route is 0.4 mile longer it is much more scenic.

Choosing the left course, you climb fairly steeply through a mountain-hemlock forest before arriving at the open expanse of Sunshine Meadows and a four-way junction with the Pacific Crest Trail. To the left is the return route of the loop, to the right (south) is your current route, and straight ahead is an old trail that goes through a lovely meadow topped by the summits of North and Middle Sister. Since the mountain views from this meadow are partially obstructed, consider making a fun side trip on this old trail past campsites and up a steep rocky slope to a small plateau featuring tiny Arrowhead Lake and more open views.

Heading south n the PCT, a quick examination of the rocks underfoot reveals why the entry route is called the *Obsidian* Trail and why walking barefoot here is not recommended. The black glass rock chips can be razor-sharp.

You hike past a gushing spring and then drop to joyful Obsidian Falls (which makes for a *very* cold shower) and a junction. Keep left (south) on the PCT and soon leave the dayhikers behind.

After 2 miles from Obsidian Falls, turn right at a junction and descend sometimes steeply to the north end of beautiful Linton Meadows. This large wildflower garden is one of the trip's many highlights. A lovely clear creek cascades down from springs and then crosses this grassy expanse. Middle Sister, South Sister, and The Husband surround the basin, providing unequalled mountain views. The meadow is popular with backpackers, so consider hiking northwest for 1.0 mile to tiny Eileen Lake for the night.

Tip: The best views from this pool are from the trailless northwest shore.

To continue your tour, pass the south end of Linton Meadows with its unique view of Middle Sister (a nearly perfect, unbroken cone from this angle) before reaching rather barren Racetrack Meadows and a five-way junction.

Tip: A nice side trip from here goes down a gully to the south on an unmarked but easy-to-follow use path for 0.8 mile to large Separation Creek Meadow, with another nice creek and more views.

The main route goes left through Racetrack Meadows, sometimes following posts, back to the PCT. Turn south as the trail gradually climbs through an attractive mix of open woods and small, rolling meadows with occasional views. You pass a seasonal pond on the left, then continue on a rolling descent to Mesa Creek (good camps).

Tip: As you switchback up the slope south of this stream be sure to look back for a nice view of redheaded South Sister—the mountain is topped by reddish cinders.

Top out at a saddle and then pass through a barren flat nestled between Rock Mesa lava flow and the remains of a craggy mountain called The Wife. Eventually our trail reaches the edge of Wickiup Plain, a large, flat, almost treeless expanse of volcanic pumice. As you continue south there are ever improving views across Wickiup Plain and Rock Mesa up to shining South Sister.

Near the south end of Wickiup Plain is a junction. Turn right for 0.8 mile to reach the nearest camps with water at popular Sisters Mirror Lake. The trees here have obviously grown since this lake was named, although the top of South Sister can still be seen.

Tip: Several small off-trail lakes are nearby and provide more private camping.

Returning to the Wickiup Plain junction, go east along the meadow's south edge for 1.3 miles and then turn north and climb back into forest on the path to Moraine Lake.

Note: Several old trails and jeep roads cross Wickiup Plain but, unless it's foggy, it would be difficult to become lost.

At the junction with the Devil's Lake Trail from the south, energetic hikers have the option to make a difficult but highly rewarding side trip to the top of South Sister, Oregon's third highest mountain. To do so, turn left at this junction and follow a well-used boot path that climbs the mountain's south side. The route requires no technical climbing equipment or experience but should be attempted only in good weather.

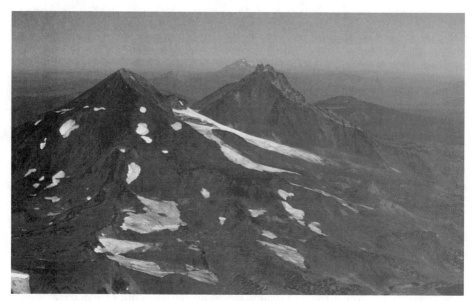

View north from summit of South Sister

Continuing on the main loop, you pass Moraine Lake (which has fair camps) and then drop through woods beside a lava flow to Fall Creek and a junction. Turn left on the popular Fall Creek Trail, which parallels its namesake stream across from the jumbled Newberry Lava Flow. After 2 miles you top out at the magnificent plain containing the Green Lakes. Nestled between South Sister and Broken Top, this basin of lakes, springs, and wildflowers is one of the most beautiful places in Oregon. Judging by the number of hikers and backpackers here, a lot of people share this opinion. Try to avoid camping here. You will, however, want to linger long enough to soak in the views and make a loop of the largest Green Lake.

Continuing north, pass to the left of the final Green Lake and begin climbing out of the basin. A long switchback and well-graded trail lead to a high, windy saddle and the start of a long drop to the east.

Tip: A worthwhile but easy-to-miss side trip is the 0.6-mile unsigned path leading south to Golden Lake. This little jewel sits in a beautiful meadow basin and features a superb view of Broken Top. The route starts about 0.9 mile beyond the pass.

The descent ends at Park Meadow, yet another remarkable spot in this wilderness. A clear creek runs through this meadow with its picturesque islands of trees, its small ponds, and its particularly photogenic view of Broken Top.

Warning: Horse packers commonly use this meadow, so the drinking water is polluted.

Tip: The best photograph here is about 100 yards upstream from the trail crossing of Park Creek.

There are numerous camps here, although they are overused, and fires are prohibited.

To continue your loop trip, head north from the meadow, following signs to Pole Creek.

Tip: Shortly after crossing the west fork of Park Creek look for an unsigned side path to the left that goes to Red Meadow. Although not as scenic as Park Meadow, it is less crowded and well worth a visit.

You top a small rise and then drop through forest to a fork of Squaw Creek. Over the next low ridge is another branch of Squaw Creek—this one dirty with glacial silt. After another 0.7 mile of uneventful hiking, you reach the welcome banks of Soap Creek and a trail junction. Good campsites are available in the nearby trees.

Two outstanding side trips leave the main loop at this point. If the weather is good, try to make time for both of them. The first climbs the 5-mile trail to Camp Lake and the Chambers Lakes.

Warning: Beware of a tricky crossing of Squaw Creek—particularly on warm afternoons with lots of glacial melting above.

A night spent at popular Camp Lake is likely to be cold and windy, but will be richly rewarded with terrific scenery. If the weather is good, I highly recommend carrying your gear up here and spending the night. From Camp Lake you could also take an extra day to scramble up the steep, rocky south slope of Middle Sister to its summit. This climb is recommended only for confident and experienced hikers.

The second side trip from the Soap Creek crossing is less crowded and visits no lakes but is still glorious. Follow an unmarked use path up the north bank of Soap Creek. After about 3 miles you'll reach a large, flat pumice meadow beneath the towering cliffs on the east face of North Sister. This is a spectacular spot although, like Camp Lake, it's too exposed for comfortable camping in bad weather.

The sometimes dusty main loop trail continues north from Soap Creek for 0.6 mile to a junction with the Pole Creek Trail and then takes a rather monotonous course through dry, mostly viewless terrain for 5.7 miles to a junction with the Scott Trail.

Tip: *A fine way to break up this segment is to follow a faint use path up splashing Alder Creek to its highly scenic headwaters beneath the northeast side of North Sister.*

Turn left at the Scott Trail junction and climb for 1.8 miles to Scott Pass where there is a junction with the Pacific Crest Trail beside tiny South Matthieu Lake. The three designated camps here are justifiably popular with both weekend backpackers and PCT through hikers.

Tip 1: *Excellent short evening strolls lead to high points both north and south of this pool. Both are terrific places to watch the sunset.*

Tip 2: *If the weather is threatening, more sheltered camps are available at North Matthieu Lake.*

Your loop trip is nearly complete now, but the remaining hike is *not* an anticlimax. Ahead lie still more grand scenery and the most interesting geology of the tour. Walk south on the PCT, cross a short section of lava, and then round the slopes of a relatively recent cinder cone called Yapoah Crater. Another 0.6 mile leads to a junction in a meadow that in early to mid-August is filled with blue lupine blossoms. You gradually climb past tiny Minnie Scott Spring (which has fair camps) and then go back into the lava to oddly named Opie Dilldock Pass.

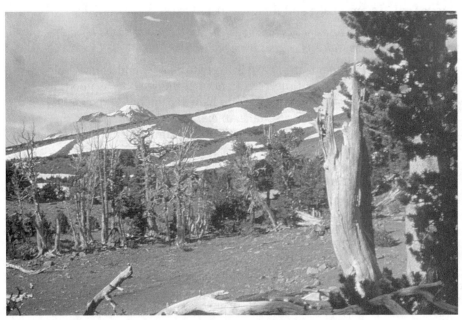

South Sister from Soap Creek headwaters

From here a not-to-be-missed side trip climbs to Collier Glacier Viewpoint. As the name advertises, this spot provides an excellent view of this massive ice sheet, one of the largest in Oregon.

Back on the PCT, travel south through a lava flow to a crossing of White Branch Creek, the outflow of Collier Glacier. An up-and-down hike, mostly in forest, leads to the junction in Sunshine Meadows you hit on day one. Turn right and follow the Obsidian Trail 4.8 miles back to your car. The hike may now be behind you, but expect the memories to last forever.

POSSIBLE ITINERARY			
	Camp	Miles	Elevation Gain
Day 1	Eileen Lake	10.6	2100
Day 2	Sisters Mirror Lake	12.3	1500
Day 3	Park Meadow	12.9	1700
Day 4	Camp Lake	8.8	1800
Day 5	Soap Creek (with side trip up Soap Creek)	11.6	1300
Day 6	South Matthieu Lake	7.5	1300
Day 7	Out	11.3	900

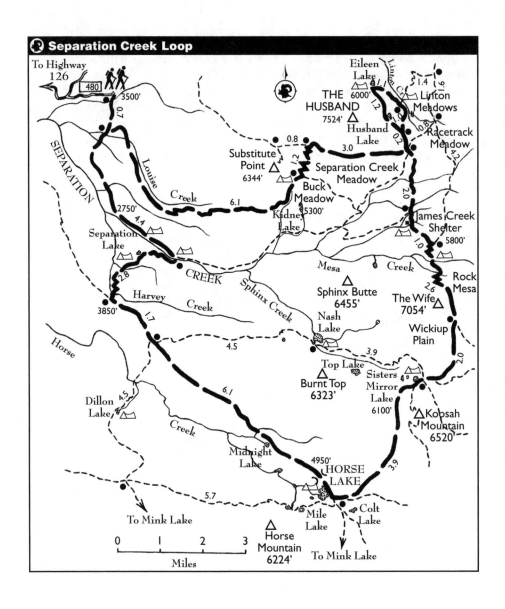

To Highway
126
480
3500'

0.7

SEPARATION

Louise

Creek

2750'
4.4

Separation
Lake

2.8

Harvey   Creek

3850'
1.7

Horse

Dillon   4.5
Lake

Creek

Midnight
Lake

CREEK

Sphinx Creek

4.5

6.1

5.7

To Mink Lake

0   1   2   3
Miles

Eileen
Lake
6000'

THE
HUSBAND
7524'

Husband
Lake

0.8

Substitute
Point
6344'

Separation Creek
Meadow

Buck
Meadow
5300'

Kidney
Lake

Mesa   Creek

Sphinx Butte
6455'

Nash
Lake

Top Lake

Burnt Top
6323'

Sisters
Mirror
Lake
6100'

Mesa

Linton

1.4

Linton
Meadows

0.8

Racetrack
Meadow

3.0   0.2

2.0

4.2

James Creek
Shelter
5800'

1.0

Rock
Mesa
2.6

The Wife
7054'

Wickiup
Plain

2.0

3.9

Koosah
Mountain
6520'

4950'
HORSE
LAKE

3.9

Colt
Lake

Mile
Lake

Horse
Mountain
6224'

To Mink Lake

10 Separation Creek Loop

RATINGS (1–10)			MILES	ELEVATION GAIN	DAYS	SHUTTLE MILEAGE
Scenery	Solitude	Difficulty				
6	7	6	42	4700	4–6	N/A
			(44)	(5200)	(4–6)	

MAP Geographics—*Three Sisters Wilderness*

USUALLY OPEN Mid-July to October

BEST Mid-July to October

PERMIT Yes (free at the trailhead)

RULES Maximum group size of 12 people; no fires near Sisters Mirror, Eileen, or Husband lakes; no camping within 100 feet of trails or water in Linton Meadows and around Eileen and Husband lakes

CONTACT McKenzie River Ranger District, (541) 822-3381

SPECIAL ATTRACTIONS Solitude; wildflowers; mountain meadows

PROBLEMS Mosquitoes until about mid-August

HOW TO GET THERE From Eugene, drive 53 miles east on State Highway 126 to a junction with Forest Road 2643 exactly 0.6 mile past the McKenzie River Ranger Station. Turn right (south) and go 7.7 miles on this one-lane paved road to a junction where the pavement ends. Veer right, drive 0.6 mile, and then bear right onto Forest Road 480 and proceed 1.2 miles to the Separation Lake Trailhead.

INTRODUCTION The Three Sisters Wilderness is the most visited wilderness area in Oregon, so it's not surprising that hikers sometimes have a hard time finding uncrowded trails. But solitude-loving pedestrians need not fear because such trails do exist. The key to finding them is to realize that the vast majority of the visitors to this huge wilderness concentrate around a handful of very popular destinations. If you avoid these areas, there is a good chance you will have the trail all to yourself. This loop takes you through some of the quietest parts of the preserve as it makes a long, woodsy approach to the more crowded high country. In addition to solitude, this warm-up period helps build anticipation for the great scenery to come and, if you start your trip on a Saturday, as most people do, it won't be until the quieter days of mid-week that you reach the popular meadows and lakes around timberline.

DESCRIPTION The trail begins in a stately old-growth forest dominated by western hemlocks and Douglas firs mixed with a few western red cedars and Pacific yews. After 0.7 mile of minor ups and downs, you reach a junction and the start of the loop.

For the recommended counterclockwise tour, go straight on the Separation Lake Trail, which over the next mile crosses four branches of Louise Creek, the third and largest branch on a convenient log. The sometimes brushy trail then contours through viewless but attractive woods for about 1 mile before gradually descending to the bottom of the heavily forested canyon of Separation Creek. From here, the trail follows this cascading creek upstream for 1.2 miles to an excellent campsite and then gradually ascends another 0.8 mile to a second campsite and a junction.

The trail that goes straight at this junction receives only limited maintenance and has been closed in recent years by blowdown. So, turn right, cross the creek on a flat-topped log, and then traverse the slope on the south side of the stream. The next 1.1 miles take you gently uphill to lily-pad-filled Separation Lake, which is surrounded by skunk-cabbage bogs and dense forests and has a good campsite above its southeastern shore. About 0.5 mile beyond Separation Lake you cross an unnamed creek and then make a very steep 700-foot climb of a wooded slope. At the top of the climb you step over tiny Harvey Creek and come to a junction. Turn left on Horse Creek Trail and ascend this gently graded route for 1.6 miles to an easily missed junction. For a really long loop you could turn right, walk past seldom-visited Dillon Lake, and then continue about 12 miles south to the Mink Lake Basin. From there, you would turn north on the Pacific Crest Trail and return to the main loop near Horse Lake.

Instead, the recommended trail goes straight at the faint junction and, 0.1 mile later, reaches a fork and another choice of routes. The shorter option goes left on the Nash Lake Trail, which passes its name-sake lake after 4.5 miles and then climbs to a junction with the PCT near Sisters Mirror Lake. The other option is slightly longer but is recommended because it is more scenic. For this alternative, go right at the fork and begin a mostly forested climb. After 3.5 pleasant but uneventful miles the trail levels off near small Midnight Lake. The trail then contours for 2 miles along a ridge on the north side of the Horse Creek valley. Shortly after it goes through an indistinct pass, the trail reaches a series of excellent campsites beside large and popular Horse Lake.

Tip: For even better campsites, take the rugged angler's path that loops around the west side of this scenic lake.

Warning: In July, the mosquitoes are voracious around Horse Lake and often seem to rival in size the lake's namesake animal.

At the east end of Horse Lake is a junction. Bear left on a dusty trail and walk uphill for 0.2 mile to a second junction. Turn left (north) and go steadily uphill through viewless forest for 3 rather monotonous miles to a group of small lakes and ponds on the meadowy Sisters Mirror Plateau. There are several enchanting heather-rimmed pools here, almost all of which feature good campsites, although fires are prohibited. In the middle of this plateau you merge with the PCT just before reaching Sisters Mirror Lake. The view from here of South Sister, which the lake once "mirrored," is now mostly obstructed by trees, but this popular lake is still very beautiful.

Tip: The campsites at Sisters Mirror Lake are often crowded. For more privacy, consider going to any of several off-trail lakes to the west.

A little past Sisters Mirror Lake is a junction with the Nash Lake Trail, where you connect with the shorter loop option discussed earlier. Go straight and walk 0.3 mile to the next junction, where you bear left, staying on the PCT. From here, make a brief traverse through woods before crossing the west side of Wickiup Plain, a large and sparsely vegetated pumice-covered meadow. This plain provides excellent views of bulky South Sister and the large obsidian, lava, and pumice flow called Rock Mesa spread out at the mountain's base. To the northeast is Middle Sister, a sharp pyramid that rises a little to the left of her taller southern sibling. In keeping with the area's family theme, the small rocky peak on the left (northwest) side of Wickiup Plain is called The Wife.

At the north end of Wickiup Plain is a junction. Go straight, traverse a waterless depression just below the edge of Rock Mesa, and then descend two switchbacks to an excellent campsite near the second of two branches of spring-fed Mesa Creek. The trail almost immediately climbs away from Mesa Creek, gaining about 200 feet to a junction. The PCT goes straight, but for this trip turn sharply left, following signs to Linton Meadows, and wander up and down through open forest and past small meadows for 0.8 mile to James Creek Shelter. This well-maintained wooden structure is an excellent place to camp because it has water and boasts a fine view of the top third of South Sister over a lush little meadow.

About 0.2 mile past the shelter you hop over tiny Hinton Creek and immediately reach a junction. Go straight, soon cross Separation Creek

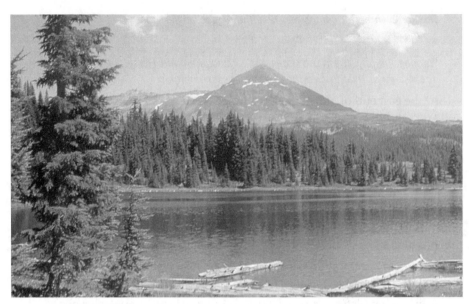

Middle Sister over Eileen Lake

on a log, and then make a 2-mile traverse that ends at a confusing junction at the southwestern tip of pumice-covered Racetrack Meadow. The unsigned trail that goes sharply left leads in less than 1 mile to Separation Creek Meadow, a worthwhile side trip for its flowers and nice view of Middle Sister. The main trail, however, goes straight at the Separation Creek Meadow junction and, 20 yards later, reaches a signed four-way junction.

The Foley Ridge Trail, which goes left here, is the return route of this loop. Before going that way, however, take the scenic side trip to Linton Meadows and Eileen Lake. So go straight, walk 0.2 mile across the west side of Racetrack Meadow, and then come to a fork. This junction is the start of a very scenic loop. Bear right (slightly downhill) and descend past great viewpoints of Middle Sister's nearly perfect pyramid to the green, flowery wonderland of Linton Meadows. The beauty of this oasis is enhanced by spring-fed Linton Creek, which tumbles down a tiered waterfall to the east before meandering across the meadow. Towering above the flower-studded grassland are Middle Sister, South Sister, and The Husband all vying for the title of being the most beautiful member of their extended family. It's a tough contest to judge, and one on which you can spend several happy hours trying to make up your mind. Camping is not allowed within 100 feet of water or trails in Linton Meadows.

At the north end of Linton Meadows are some possible campsites and a junction. Bear left and make a scenic 1.1-mile jaunt to spectacular Eileen Lake. This small meadow-rimmed gem has very scenic (but overused) campsites and, from the northwestern shore, views of the Three Sisters that will take your breath away. Fires are prohibited within 0.25 mile of this lake as well as at nearby Husband Lake.

From the outlet of Eileen Lake the trail turns south and goes gradually uphill to Husband Lake. From the east (nontrail) side of this shallow lake there are stunning reflections of (appropriately enough) The Husband. A little beyond Husband Lake you close the side-trip loop when you reach the junction with the trail to Linton Meadows. Go straight to return to the junction with the Foley Ridge Trail at the southwest corner of Racetrack Meadow.

Go right (west) and travel gently up and down for 3 miles through forest and past several stagnant ponds to a junction. Turn left and descend a half-dozen switchbacks to a junction at the north end of long and narrow Buck Meadow. The well-used trail that goes straight dead-ends after 100 yards at a leaky wooden shelter and a possible campsite.

Warning: The tiny creek here usually dries up by late summer.

Your trail, which is very faint at first, veers right at the junction and travels along the west side of grassy, 0.5-mile-long Buck Meadow. From the south end of the meadow, the trail makes a brief climb to the west and then begins a long descent. The entire route is through forest, which becomes increasingly lush with a denser understory as you lose elevation. A little over 6 miles from Buck Meadow is the junction with the Separation Lake Trail and the close of the loop. Turn right and thus back to your car.

POSSIBLE ITINERARY

	Camp	Miles	Elevation Gain
Day 1	Separation Lake	6.2	200
Day 2	Horse Lake	9.4	1800
Day 3	James Creek Shelter	9.6	1700
Day 4	Eileen Lake (with side trip to Separation Creek Meadow)	6.3	800
Day 5	Out	12.4	700

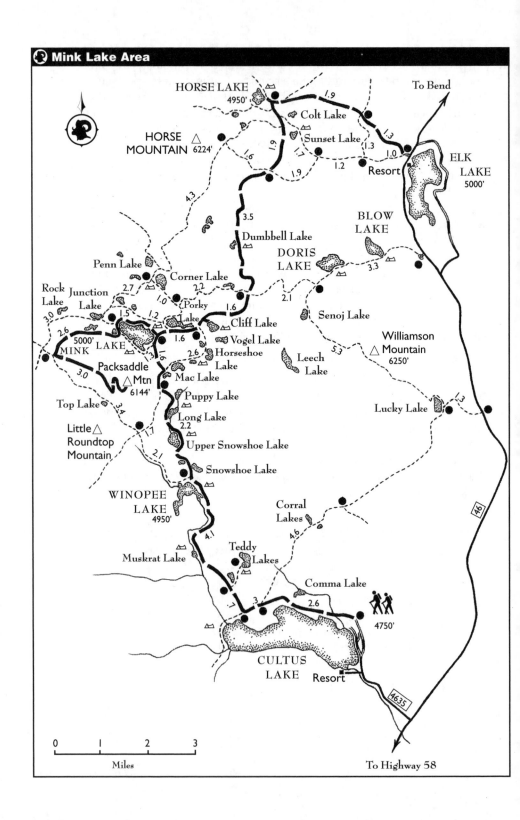

11 Mink Lake Area

RATINGS (1–10)			MILES	ELEVATION GAIN	DAYS	SHUTTLE MILEAGE
Scenery	Solitude	Difficulty				
7	4	3	24	1600	3	16
			(38)	(3300)	(3–5)	

MAP Geographics—*Three Sisters Wilderness*

USUALLY OPEN July to October

BEST Late August to September

PERMITS Yes

RULES No camping or fires within 100 feet of lakes

CONTACT Bend/Fort Rock Ranger District, (541) 383-4000

SPECIAL ATTRACTIONS Fishing and swimming lakes; relatively easy hiking

PROBLEMS Mosquitoes in July and early August; crowded in spots

HOW TO GET THERE For a south-to-north tour start from the east end of Cultus Lake. Drive State Highway 372 and Road 46 (the "Many Lakes Highway") either 44 miles west and south from Bend or 27 miles north from the Highway 58 turnoff near Crescent Lake. From near the north end of Crane Prairie Reservoir, turn west on Road 4635 to Cultus Lake. At a fork keep right toward the campground and then right again on dirt Road 100 to its end at the trailhead. The north trailhead is just off Road 46, 31 miles west of Bend, across from the Elk Lake Resort.

INTRODUCTION The south half of the Three Sisters Wilderness has a totally different character than the north. There are no tall peaks, no glaciers, few meadows, and only limited views. What the hiker will discover, however, are miles of pleasant forest trails and enough lakes to impress even Minnesota natives. Every turn of the trail seems to reveal another lovely mountain pool ranging from a small pond to a large lake. Each is different enough in character that lovers of lake fishing, swimming, rafting, or just viewing can stay happy for weeks. The second nice thing about this country is the easy hiking. Since almost everything is at roughly the same elevation, extended ups and downs simply

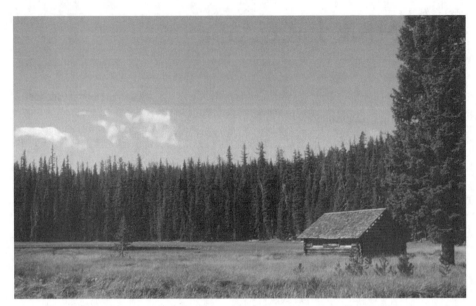

Muskrat Lake with a nearby old trapper's cabin

don't exist—which means a lot less work for tired backpackers. This trip is perfect for hikers of advancing years with knees that suffer on long downhills or as a first long backpack for younger travelers. Easy trails and numerous lakes allow for short hiking days and lots of time for lazy afternoons.

All that water, of course, has one big drawback—*mosquitoes!* The clouds of flying vampires here are thicker than a Dairy Queen milkshake. In July your essential gear should include repellent, a headnet, and an extra pint or two of blood to replace that stolen by the bugs. Fortunately, by mid-August or so the number of invertebrates has dropped dramatically, and by September you can comfortably travel without repellent or even a tent—the rain gods permitting, of course.

DESCRIPTION   From the Cultus Lake Trailhead, hike west along the lakeshore path, passing several good swimming beaches with views across this large lake. The trail veers away from the lake after 1.7 miles and leads northwest for 0.9 mile to a junction with the trail to Corral Lakes. Go straight here and 0.3 mile farther turn right at a second junction. After 0.7 mile, you pass the side trail to the Teddy Lakes (which has good camps). Another 1.4 miles of easy walking leads to the lovely meadow holding lily-pad-filled Muskrat Lake with its quaint little cabin. Take time to visit this comfortable cabin, which is open to the public for overnight use on a first-come, first-served basis. More good camps are available in the woods at the lake's north end near the inlet creek.

Muskrat Lake is an inviting camp spot, but you probably won't be tired when you get there, since in 5 miles the elevation gain has been only 200 feet. With all that extra energy you might prefer to continue north to equally scenic Winopee Lake. The route gradually gains a bit of elevation as it parallels a small creek (usually nothing more than a trickle by late summer). About 2 miles from Muskrat Lake is the south shore of large, irregularly shaped Winopee Lake. The trail works around the east shore of this lake, mostly in viewless forest, to a lovely meadow at the north end. This meadow is well worth exploring, although it's rather boggy.

At the trail junction beside Winopee Lake keep right and in rapid succession reach Snowshoe Lake and two smaller, unnamed lakes, as you *slowly* climb on this attractive route. Upper Snowshoe Lake is the next highlight, with its excellent camps and lunch spots. Here, as at all the larger lakes along this tour, the hiker should look for goldeneye (a duck), osprey, and bald eagles—all common in the area. Continuing your hike north, the seemingly endless parade of lovely lakes continues with Long Lake and Puppy Lake. At a meadow holding Desane Lake is a junction with the Pacific Crest Trail. Turn right on the PCT to reach the shores of S Lake and another junction.

The PCT keeps right here, passing yet another string of attractive lakes. The recommended route, however, turns left, climbs a low ridge, and then drops fairly steeply into the basin containing popular Mink Lake. Dozens of excellent camps surround this scenic 360-acre lake. The best views are from the northeast shore near an old shelter. Good camps and worthwhile dayhike destinations are

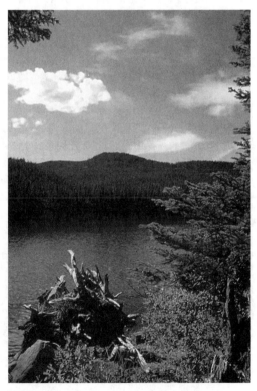

Packsaddle Mountain over Mink Lake

found in almost every direction. The author's favorite camps are a little to the east at Porky Lake, but other nearby lakes (some off-trail) provide more private locations.

A highly recommended dayhike side trip is the path from Mink Lake to the top of Packsaddle Mountain, the area's highest viewpoint. The climb is fairly long but worthwhile, and the tired hiker can look forward to returning to a lakeside camp and a pleasant swim. The path starts from near Junction Lake west of Mink Lake. Some of the less strenuous dayhike options include Corner Lake, Junction Lake, and Cabin Meadows.

To continue the recommended trip, hike along the south side of Porky Lake and then climb out of the lakes basin back to the PCT. Turn north and after about 100 yards reach the possibly unsigned 0.1-mile side trail to Cliff Lake.

> **Tip:** Be sure to visit this scenic lake since it features good camps, a trail shelter, and great diving rocks along the north shore.

The PCT continues north and east through forests and meadows. You pass several small rock formations on the way to a four-way junction with the Six Lakes Trail. Keep straight (north) on the PCT along an easy route through rolling mountain-hemlock forests. The trail passes tiny Island Lake and larger Dumbbell Lake (good camps) and then drops

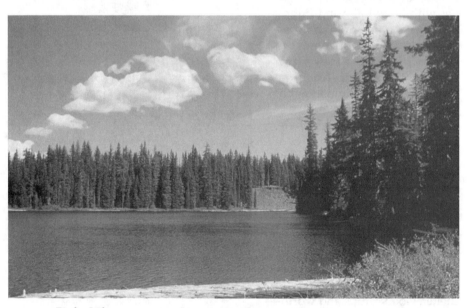

Porky Lake

over a gentle saddle to a four-way junction west of Island Meadow. If the weather is bad, turn right here for a quick exit back to the Elk Lake Trailhead. Otherwise, veer left to reach Horse Lake—just 2 miles away.

Horse Lake is the largest and prettiest of another cluster of lakes. Excellent campsites abound near Horse Lake, but for more privacy try nearby Mile or Park Lake.

Tip 1: The best lunch spot at Horse Lake is on the rock peninsula on the lake's west shore—reached by an angler's path around the lake. The view from here includes a nice perspective of Mount Bachelor.

Tip 2: If you have an extra day and good route finding skills, consider visiting Burnt Top. Take the trail going northwest from Horse Lake for about 1.8 miles and then hope to find the unmaintained 3.5-mile route to the right leading to Burnt Top's summit views.

To return to your car, head due east from Horse Lake on well-used Trail #3516. You gradually climb to a viewless pass and a junction with the PCT. Keep straight on a dusty trail and in 1.3 miles reach civilization, in the form of the Elk Lake Trailhead.

POSSIBLE ITINERARY			
	Camp	Miles	Elevation Gain
Day 1	Mink Lake	11.5	500
Day 2	Mink Lake (day trip up Packsaddle Mountain)	14.0	1700
Day 3	Horse Lake	8.8	700
Day 4	Out	3.4	400

Note: For loop lovers, this area provides several possible options. One alternative is to start your trip at the Lucky Lake Trailhead. Hike southwest via Corral Lakes to Cultus Lake, turn north past Winopee and Mink lakes to the Six Lakes Trail, and then return via Senoj Lake and Williamson Mountain.

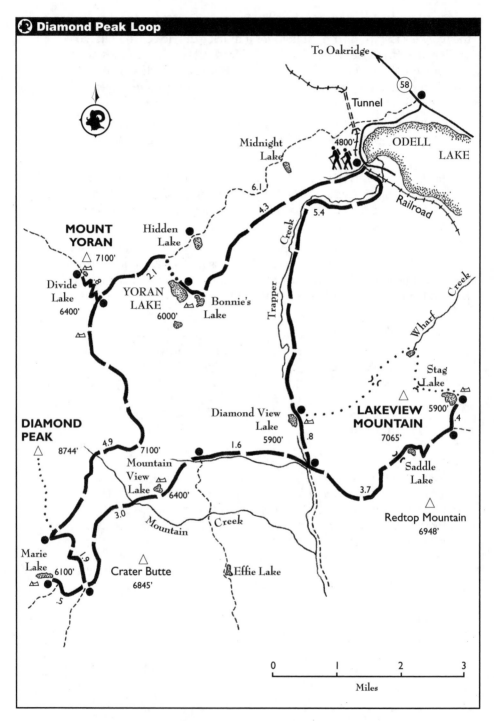

To Oakridge

58

Tunnel

Midnight
Lake

4800'

ODELL

LAKE

6.1

4.3

5.4

Railroad

MOUNT
YORAN

△ 7100'

Hidden
Lake

2.1

Divide
Lake
6400'

YORAN
LAKE
6000'

Bonnie's
Lake

Trapper

Creek

Wharf

Creek

Stag
Lake

LAKEVIEW
MOUNTAIN
7065'

Diamond View
Lake
5900'

5900'

.4

DIAMOND
PEAK

△ 8744'

4.9

7100'

1.6

.8

Mountain
View
Lake
6400'

3.0

Mountain

Creek

1.9

Saddle
Lake

3.7

Redtop Mountain
6948'

Marie
Lake
6100'

.5

△
Crater Butte
6845'

Effie Lake

0   1   2   3

Miles

12 Diamond Peak Loop

RATINGS (1–10)			MILES	ELEVATION GAIN	DAYS	SHUTTLE MILEAGE
Scenery	Solitude	Difficulty				
8	6	5	27	3500	3–4	N/A
			(36)	(4300)	(4–5)	

MAP   USFS—*Diamond Peak Wilderness*

USUALLY OPEN   July to October

BEST   Mid- to late July

PERMITS   Yes

RULES   Group size limited to 12 persons

CONTACT   Crescent Ranger District, (541) 433-3200

SPECIAL ATTRACTIONS   Relative solitude; scenic lakes; relatively easy loop

PROBLEMS   Mosquitoes

HOW TO GET THERE   Follow Highway 58 southeast from Eugene for 70 miles to Willamette Pass. Just east of the pass turn right on West Odell Lake Road. Follow this paved route for 1.8 miles to the well-marked Yoran Lake Trailhead.

INTRODUCTION   The high, snowy ridge of Diamond Peak rises impressively over the lush forests and quiet lakes south of Willamette Pass. Despite easy access and beautiful scenery, the wilderness surrounding this mountain receives less use than other areas. Like a neglected stepchild, Diamond Peak is ignored by most Oregonians in favor of the Three Sisters to the north or Mount Thielsen to the south. Diamond Peak, however, provides scenery to rival any other major Cascade peak—and this trip proves it.

DESCRIPTION   To hike this loop counterclockwise, take the trail to Yoran Lake. Climb gradually through generally viewless forests for 4 miles to irregularly shaped Bonnie's Lake and larger Yoran Lake just beyond. There are good campsites at both lakes, but Yoran Lake has the edge in

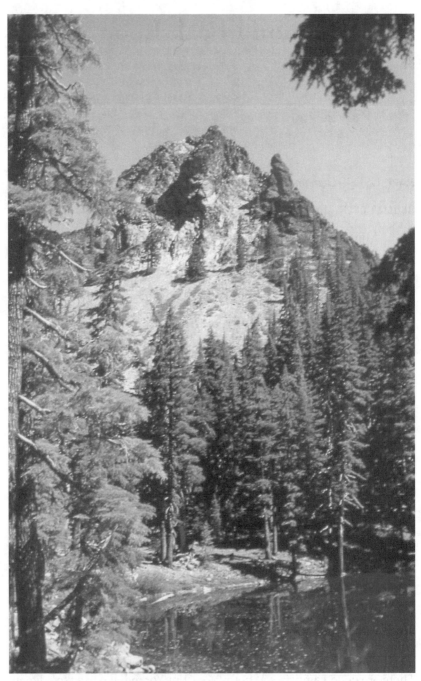

Mount Yoran over Divide Lake

Backpacking Oregon

scenery since it boasts a forested island and a good, if partly obstructed, view of Diamond Peak.

Hike around to the north end of Yoran Lake and then break out the compass and climb cross-country on a northwest course through forests for about 0.4 mile to the Pacific Crest Trail. Turn left and follow this well-graded route to a junction with the trail to Divide Lake. For a side trip and campsite turn right, climb over a low saddle, and switchback down to Divide Lake. The towering double summits of Mount Yoran loom over the north shore of this deep little pool.

Tip: Don't forget your wide-angle lens.

Nearby small ponds and heather meadows add to the magic of this scene. The best camps here are at the west end of the lake.

Tip: A superior late-afternoon or evening stroll follows the trail along a ridge northwest of Divide Lake. After about 0.5 mile there is a terrific view of Diamond Peak.

Now return to the Pacific Crest Trail and turn south. This scenic route soon passes a pair of lovely ponds with a nearby campsite, climbs a bit, and then begins a long contour across the view-packed meadows and talus slopes on the east shoulder of Diamond Peak. The route is very scenic and very high. Be prepared to cross snowfields here through July.

An exceptional side trip for fit and experienced hikers is the steep cross-country scramble to the summit of Diamond Peak. After the trail begins to descend from the high country, leave the PCT just before a switchback on the south side of the peak and scramble up the long south ridge. The route is exposed and rocky and should be attempted only in good weather, but it does not require technical climbing skill or equipment. On a clear day the view from atop Diamond Peak may be the best in Oregon. From here you can see all the way from Mount Hood to California's Mount Shasta. To the east, stretch the seemingly endless forests and deserts of eastern Oregon.

Back on the trail, you drop through open forests to a four-way junction. To reach the good camps at quiet Marie Lake, turn right and hike 0.5 mile through a pumice meadow with nice views of Diamond Peak.

Return to the PCT junction and go straight (traveling north and east) on a sketchy route that climbs through open mountain-hemlock forests.

Tip: Watch for tree blazes to help you navigate this trail.

After 1.6 miles is a beautiful meadow where you cross Mountain Creek and then hike downhill through forest another 0.7 mile to reach shallow Mountain View Lake. The mosquitoes here are particularly fierce

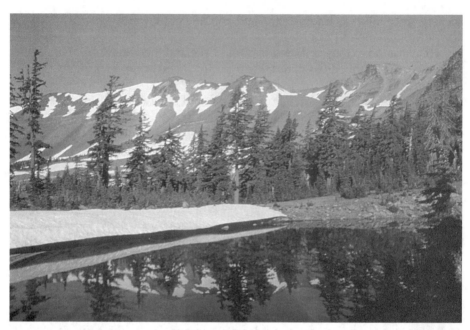

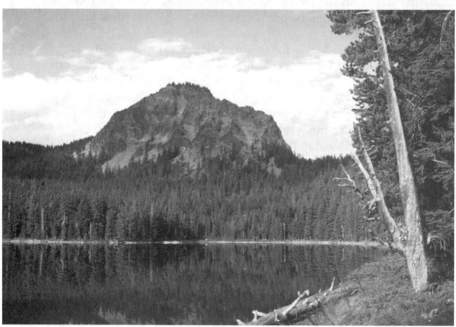

Top: *Diamond Peak over an unnamed pond, above the Pacific Crest Trail*
Bottom: *Lakeview Mountain over Stag Lake*

in July so camping is not recommended, but the reflected view of the long, snowy ridge of Diamond Peak is exceptional. Unfortunately, later in the season—when the bugs are gone—the snow on the mountain has melted and the lake's level is lower so the view isn't as good. Continue hiking east for 2.4 forested miles to a possibly dry creekbed and a four-way junction. Turn left and hike 0.8 mile to aptly named Diamond View Lake. There are several good camps at this popular and scenic lake. The bugs here are less numerous than at Mountain View Lake, but you'll still be glad you brought repellent and a tent with mosquito netting.

A highly recommended side trip starts from the junction south of Diamond View Lake. Go east and climb gradually to a pass containing appropriately named Saddle Lake and then continue another 1.3 miles to reach the side trail to Stag Lake. Turn left to reach this shallow pool with its excellent camps and a superb view of the cliffs on the east face of Lakeview Mountain. Hikers accomplished with a map and compass can scramble steeply over a pass west of Stag Lake and drop to a secluded pool north of Lakeview Mountain. There are great views of this craggy butte from the pool's north shore. Now you travel south-west past another pond and through yet another saddle before striking off west by southwest to reach the trail near Diamond View Lake. The entire circuit of Lakeview Mountain makes for a challenging but highly satisfying day trip from a base camp at Diamond View Lake.

To complete the trip, you hike north from Diamond View Lake through monotonous lodgepole-pine forests. On the left, rushing Trapper Creek plays hide and seek with the trail for a few miles before you finally cross it and make the short jog back to your car.

POSSIBLE ITINERARY

	Camp	Miles	Elevation Gain
Day 1	Divide Lake	7.3	2100
Day 2	Marie Lake	8.1	800
Day 3	Diamond View Lake	5.9	500
Day 4	Diamond View Lake (day trip to Stag Lake)	9.8	800
Day 5	Out	5.4	100

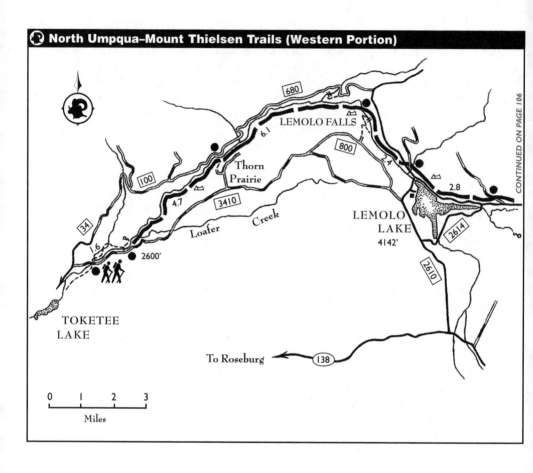

CONTINUED ON PAGE 106

680

LEMOLO FALLS

6.1

800

.4

100

Thorn
Prairie

2.8

34

4.7

3410

Loafer   Creek

LEMOLO
LAKE
4142'

2614

.6

2600'

2610

TOKETEE
LAKE

To Roseburg   138

0   1   2   3
Miles

13   North Umpqua– Mount Thielsen Trails

RATINGS (1–10)			MILES	ELEVATION GAIN	DAYS	SHUTTLE MILEAGE
Scenery	Solitude	Difficulty				
7	6	6	46	6800	4–5	34
			(48)	(8700)	(4–6)	

MAP   USFS—*Umpqua National Forest & Mount Thielsen Wilderness*

USUALLY OPEN   Late June to October

BEST   July

PERMITS   None

RULES   Maximum group size of 12 persons; no camping within 100 feet of lakes

CONTACT   Diamond Lake Ranger District, (541) 498-2531

SPECIAL ATTRACTIONS   Waterfalls; mountain scenery; diverse landscapes; easy road access

PROBLEMS   Unattractive section near Lemolo Lake; mosquitoes at higher elevations in July; long stretches without water

HOW TO GET THERE   The end of this hike is easy to locate. Drive Highway 138 east from the Crater Lake entrance road to the marked Pacific Crest Trail parking area. The starting point is trickier to locate. From Highway 138 about 20 miles west of Diamond Lake (or 57 miles east of Roseburg), turn north on paved Road 34, signed as the Toketee—Rigdon Road. After about 200 yards keep left and cross the river, staying on Road 34. Drive for 2 miles and then turn right on gravel Road 3401 (Thorn Prairie Road). After 2 more pothole-plagued miles pull into a parking area on the left (unsigned but built to accommodate visitors to the Umpqua Hot Springs).

> *Tip: Be especially careful to leave nothing of value in your car. Trailheads for hot springs often seem to attract burglars.*

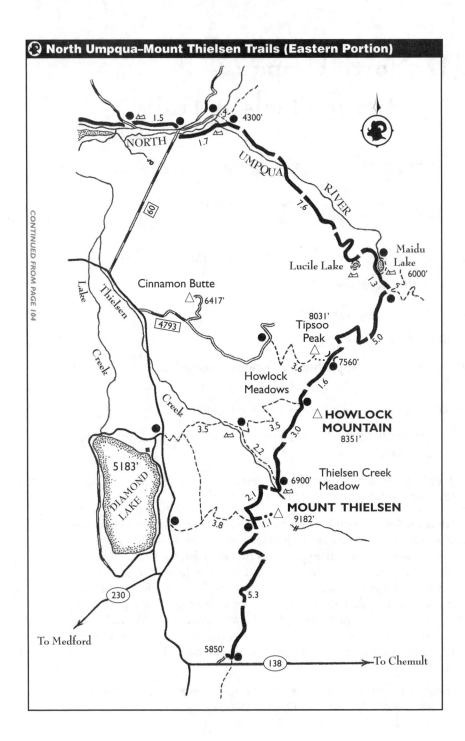

CONTINUED FROM PAGE 104

North

Umpqua River

1.5 1.4 4300' 1.7 60 7.6

Maidu Lake 6000'

Lucile Lake 1.3

Cinnamon Butte 6417' Lake Thielsen Creek 4793

8031' Tipsoo Peak 5.0 3.6 7560' 1.6

Howlock Meadows

Creek 3.5 3.5 3.0 Howlock Mountain 8351'

2.2

5183' Diamond Lake 2.1 6900' Thielsen Creek Meadow

3.5 Mount Thielsen 9182' 3.8 1.1

230

To Medford 5.3

138 5850' To Chemult

INTRODUCTION This wonderful hike has a split personality. The first part travels through the wild canyon of the North Umpqua River, where the highlights are old-growth forests, towering waterfalls, columnar basalt formations, and a lovely stream. The second half of the hike climbs to the Cascade crest and explores the scenic meadows, crags, and views around Howlock Mountain and Mount Thielsen. Few people hike these two trails in one outing because they are separated by a less attractive area around busy Lemolo Lake. Done in combination, however, they are a great experience. This is one of the few places in Oregon where it is still possible to take the long, respectful, trail approach to the high country that was formerly the only way to visit it. By starting from low-elevation riverside forests and gradually working up to the high volcanic peaks, the hiker gets a complete sampling of the Cascade Mountains' many environments and charms. It is, of course, possible to do this trip from high to low (which would mean less elevation gain), but going from low to high saves the climax scenery for the end.

Altitude is not the only difference between the two trail sections. The canyon section is a celebration of water—both in its many forms and of the beautiful things it creates. The trail passes countless large and small springs, mossy cliffs, several waterfalls, and, of course, always the enchanting river. Lush old-growth forests here feature specimens of Douglas fir, western hemlock, cedar, bigleaf maple, and Pacific yew. Ferns, mosses, and other water-loving species crowd the forest floor. In contrast to the virtual rainforest below, the high-country section of this route is amazingly dry. There is very little surface water and limited ground cover, and the forests consist of water-starved lodgepole pine and mountain hemlock. There is, of course, a reason for the striking difference between these two neighboring environments. Porous volcanic soils around Mount Thielsen allow most of the water to percolate into the ground rather than flowing on top. This water later feeds the many springs in the lower canyon. Lemolo Lake marks the dividing point between the two environments, and the change from one to the other is remarkably sudden.

Note: *If done separately, the peak seasons for the two trail sections are late May to mid-June for the lower canyon, and mid- to late July for the high country.*

Warning: *The lower part of this trail is shared with mountain bikers. In theory hikers have the right of way, but in practice those on foot are forced to get off the trail to avoid being run over.*

DESCRIPTION If you start your hike on a weekday, when the hot springs are much less crowded, consider taking the steep 0.3-mile trail to the springs. To do so, cross the river on a large bridge and then turn right and climb to your goal. Here you can relax and soak your muscles in the 100-plus°F waters. You might also elect to save this experience for when you return after the hike.

Warning: Nude bathing is the norm here. Leave the children, and your modesty, at home.

The North Umpqua River Trail begins about 100 yards up the road from the parking area and starts by dropping to the left into the trees. You cross Loafer Creek and soon reach aptly named Surprise Falls, which leaps out of the ground from a large spring directly beneath the trail. Just ahead is even more impressive Columnar Falls, where smaller springs feed a lacy waterfall that drops over a moss-covered basalt cliff. At the base of this cliff the water simply disappears back into the ground. A third waterfall, this one on a more conventional side stream, is 0.2 mile beyond Columnar Falls.

As the trail continues up the canyon it encounters numerous landslides and downed trees. Storms in 1996 caused this damage and forced an extended closure of this route as trail crews worked to clear the mess. Nice job, guys! In the wettest sections, plank boardwalks have been installed to allow a dry passage for hikers. Although the trail closely parallels the river, it is rarely level as it seems to go constantly up and down between marshy river flats and cliffs above the water. The wonderful scenery amply compensates for the sweat.

Note: Most of the North Umpqua River's water flows in a diversion canal and pipeline rather than the natural streambed. The water is taken out upstream at Lemolo Lake and feeds several electric power stations. Hikers can only imagine how beautiful this canyon must have been with a full stream.

Just 1.5 miles from the start is Michelle Creek, where the trail cuts across a series of mossy rocks, springs, and small waterfalls. Another 0.5 mile of hiking takes you to three large "nurse" logs that have fallen with their upended root systems exposed. Signs identify these giants as the "Sleeping Stooges," and each log is marked with the name of one of the famous comics. ("Larry" actually bridges the river.) Continuing upstream, several river flats make nice camps for those who got a late start.

Keep straight at the junction with the Thorn Prairie connector trail, which makes a short climb to a spur road. The main trail continues upstream through more forests. On the opposite side of the river an unobtrusive gravel road follows a section of the diversion canal. About 4.5 miles from the Thorn Prairie connector, a set of power lines leads from Lemolo generator #1 on the opposite bank. The trail continues beyond the generator for 1.4 miles to a river crossing.

The roar coming from up the canyon is Lemolo Falls. At 169 feet this enormous waterfall is one of the trip's scenic highlights.

Tip: The best views are from the south. Take the time to scramble up this bank for a few hundred yards to a trail that comes down from the right. You can follow this trail upstream to reach some wonderful views of the falls' sheer drop.

While enjoying the scene, imagine how impressive this falls must have been before most of the water was diverted!

Now cross the river on a log and begin to climb. Near the top of the ascent are some partly obstructed views of the falls.

Tip: You can scramble out to the cliff edge for a better look, but this is rather dangerous and only sure-footed hikers should try it. Hang on tightly to trees for support.

Once above the falls, the trail closely follows the river as the water cascades along and drops in a series of small but attractive falls. The forests here support lots of wildflowers in May and June. The trail slowly climbs to meet the pipes and canals of the water diversion system on the left. Small leaks give the impression of natural springs, especially since water-loving plants have colonized these human-made creeklets. Where the path leaves the canyon there is a trailhead and a bridge over the canal to a paved road.

The trail resumes on the opposite side of the road and immediately enters a different environment. The lush canyon forests are replaced by open lodge-pole-pine woods. These

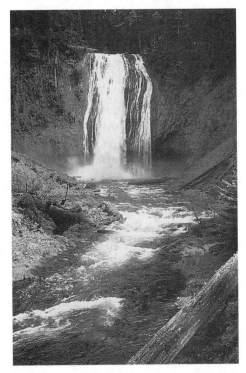

Lemolo Falls, upper North Umpqua River

trees are smaller and straighter and provide less shade than the Douglas-fir forests below. The ground cover is also more sparse and has changed from rhododendrons and ferns to huckleberries and manzanita.

The trail crosses a gravel road and a creek and then begins its long eastward course paralleling the paved road on the north side of Lemolo Lake. Occasional breaks in the trees provide views of Lemolo Lake and distant Mount Thielsen to break up the monotony. Fortunately, the trail is nearly level, so the miles go by quickly.

Tip 1: Try to do this stretch on a weekday when the road is less busy.

Tip 2: If you need water or a place to camp, simply scramble down to the lake, where there are numerous possible sites.

Presently you cross another gravel road and shortly thereafter a possibly dry creekbed.

Tip: A short side trip to the main road from here leads to a fine camp—complete with a picnic table—beside large Crystal Springs.

In another mile the trail drops to a road junction. To continue your tour, veer right, follow the road over the sparkling stream, and look for a sign on the left marking the resumption of trail. The route immediately enters wilder, more attractive terrain.

The path continues upstream for almost 2 miles before crossing the river (possible camps). Shortly thereafter is a junction with a spur trail from the Bradley Creek Campground and Trailhead. The North Umpqua River Trail turns right and begins a long, mostly viewless climb to the high country. As you gain elevation the ground cover gets more lush and the trees slowly change over to mountain hemlock. The remnants of the North Umpqua River (now only a small creek) splash along on the right. Cross the flow and begin a long sidehill climb. The trail is well graded and the route mostly in shade so the climb is not difficult. Eventually the trail turns south up a ridge, crosses a dry creekbed, and soon reaches a poorly marked trail junction.

To the right is forest-rimmed Lucile Lake. A pleasant trail circles this mountain pool where the best camps are on the southwest shore. About 0.5 mile from the Lucile Lake junction the main trail passes an excellent high viewpoint before making a short, mostly level jog to Maidu Lake. This popular lake is surrounded by forests and excellent campsites. As always, camp well away from fragile lakeshore locations.

Warning: Be prepared for lots of mosquitoes here in July.

This lake is the source of the North Umpqua River, which you have now followed upstream all the way from Umpqua Hot Springs.

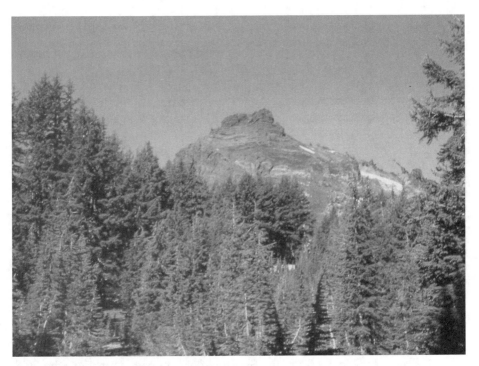

Tipsoo Peak from the Pacific Crest Trail

Tip: *Fill your water bottles here. The only trailside water for the next 11 miles is from lingering snowfields.*

To continue your tour, pass the lake and take the trail from its south end that climbs to a forested pass and a junction with the Pacific Crest Trail. Turn right and begin a long, viewless climb through mountain-hemlock forests. After 2.2 miles the trail reaches a marvelous viewpoint atop a rocky promontory. Rest and enjoy the view, and then reshoulder your pack and resume climbing. The trail circles around the remains of a flattened volcanic butte, passes another viewpoint, and comes to a saddle on the northeast side of Tipsoo Peak. Ice-age glaciers obviously ripped deeply into this reddish-colored peak's north side, although no ice remains today. You continue climbing beside a gully and then come to a meadow leading to a broad pass, where posts mark the way across a pumice-covered flat. Tired hikers rejoice—this 7,560-foot pass is the highest point on the Pacific Crest Trail in Oregon!

Tip: *Don't miss the relatively easy scramble to the excellent view atop nearby Tipsoo Peak.*

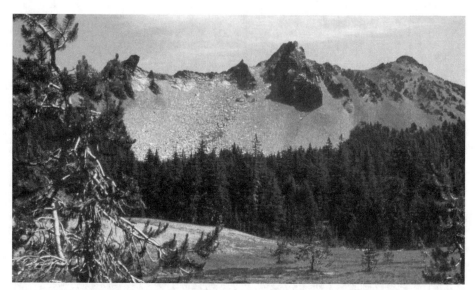

Howlock Mountain over Howlock Meadows

From the pass your trail returns to the trees and begins a gradual descent. Now you round a ridge and begin to enjoy occasional views of craggy Howlock Mountain. Shortly after you pass a junction, the PCT skirts around the left side of a large pumice flat called Howlock Meadows.

Tip: *For an exceptionally scenic view of Howlock Mountain, take the time to visit the middle of this meadow. From here it's easy to see how this section of the Cascade crest got the name "Sawtooth Ridge."*

Although camping here seems inviting, lingering snowfields provide the only water. Forced, therefore, to continue south, you can look for intermittent views of Diamond Lake and Mount Bailey to the west as you make a long, irregular descent. About 3 miles from Howlock Meadows is Thielsen Meadow and the welcome waters of Thielsen Creek. Please camp back in the trees, well away from the fragile meadows.

For several reasons Thielsen Meadow is a popular place. Water from the spring-fed stream attracts PCT hikers. Abundant wildflowers provide delicate beauty and draw their share of admirers. Most outstanding of all, however, is the jaw-dropping view of the north face of Mount Thielsen. The towering cliffs rise almost 2,300 feet above the meadow to the mountain's famous pointed summit. The incredible scenery has earned this spot a place on the author's personal list of Oregon's 10 most spectacular locations.

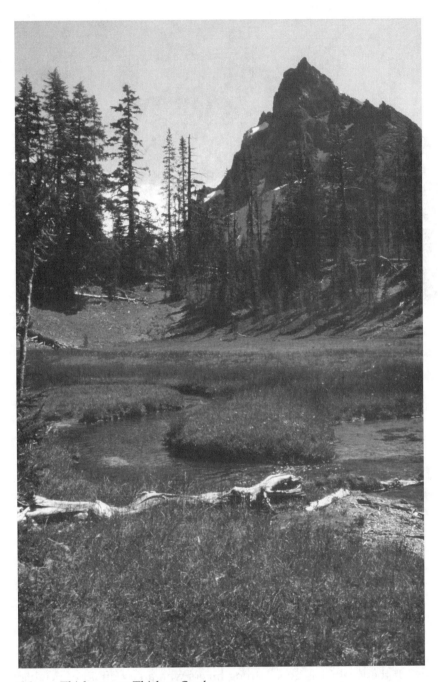

Mount Thielsen over Thielsen Creek

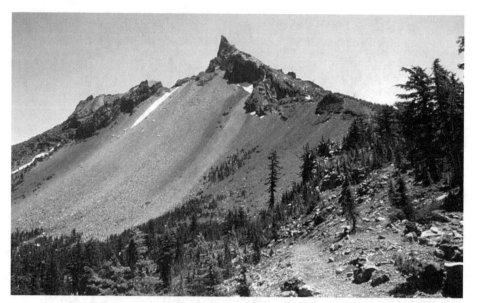

Mount Thielsen from southwest with PCT in foreground

Tip: *Photographers will need an extra-wide-angle lens to capture this scene.*

You could easily spend an extra day here just gazing up in amazement. For more exercise, venture out on any of several highly rewarding dayhikes. Nearby are the boulder field and springs at the head of Thielsen Creek and the small glacier at the base of the cliffs on the north face of Mount Thielsen. More ambitious hikers can scramble up an unnamed high point northeast of Mount Thielsen where there are outstanding views of the peak and surrounding country. A final option is to scramble over a bouldery pass to the east and then drop steeply to the huge pumice flat at the head of Cottonwood Creek, directly beneath the steep east face of Mount Thielsen.

The PCT continues south from Thielsen Creek making a long, gradual climb to a ridge where you are treated to a frontal view of the colorful scree slopes on Mount Thielsen's northwestern face. The mountain's impressive summit spire is prominently displayed. This pinnacle is a favorite target of Mother Nature's wrath, earning Mount Thielsen the nickname "Lightning Rod of the Cascades." The trail cuts across a scree slope to a second ridge where there is a junction with the Mount Thielsen Trail from Diamond Lake.

If the weather is good, strong hikers who aren't afraid of heights should take the time to climb Mount Thielsen. The unofficial trail is easy to follow as it winds through twisted mountain hemlocks and whitebark pines and passes numerous delicate rock gardens. Views of distant peaks and lakes improve with every heart-pounding step. Above the treeline the "trail" charges up a super-steep slope of scree and loose rocks, eventually topping out on a small ledge at the base of the summit pinnacle. The view from here is world class and includes most of the state of Oregon as well as parts of California. A sharp eye will even be able to see over the rim of Crater Lake not far to the south. The final 100 feet or so to the top of the mountain is definitely not for everyone. While not technically difficult, it requires using handholds and footholds to crawl carefully up the rock face. To the north and east sheer cliffs drop 2,000 to 3,000 feet, so vertigo is a real concern.

Warning: *Given this mountain's nickname, hikers should avoid this climb when there is any threat of a thunderstorm.*

After returning to the PCT, continue south and make a long, gradual, and rather uneventful descent around forested ridges to a dirt road. Cross the road and shortly thereafter turn right at a junction with the 0.2-mile trail that drops down a forested gully to the official PCT trailhead and your car.

POSSIBLE ITINERARY			
	Camp	Miles	Elevation Gain
Day 1	Below Lemolo Falls	10.6	1100
Day 2	North Umpqua crossing	9.0	900
Day 3	Maidu Lake	7.7	2100
Day 4	Thielsen Creek	10.9	2100
Day 5	Out (with side trip up Mount Thielsen)	9.6	2500

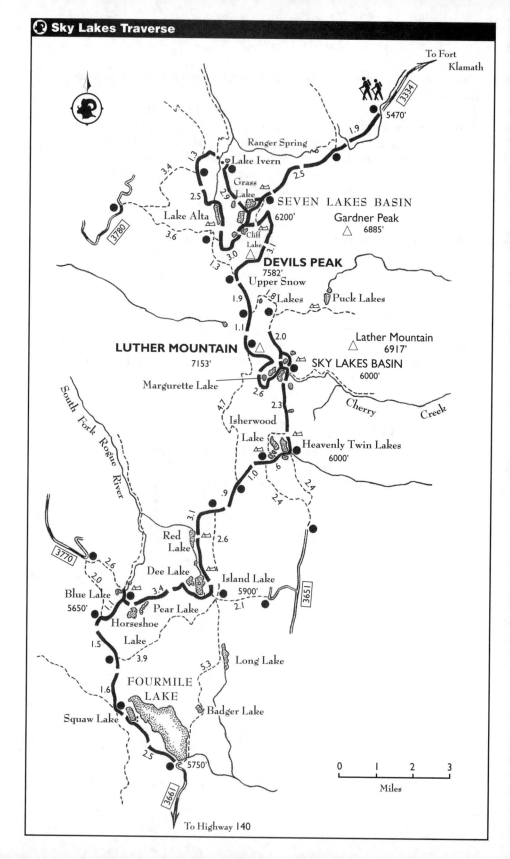

14 Sky Lakes Traverse

RATINGS (1–10)			MILES	ELEVATION GAIN	DAYS	SHUTTLE MILEAGE
Scenery	Solitude	Difficulty				
7	4	5	31 (45)	3600 (5200)	3–4 (4–6)	41

MAP USFS—*Sky Lakes Wilderness*

USUALLY OPEN July to October

BEST Mid-August to early September

PERMITS None

RULES Maximum group size of 8 people/12 stock; near lakes, camping is allowed only at designated sites

CONTACT Klamath Falls Ranger District, (541) 883-6714

SPECIAL ATTRACTIONS Huckleberries; swimming & fishing lakes

PROBLEMS Mosquitoes (through mid-August); crowded in spots

HOW TO GET THERE To reach the north trailhead, turn west off Highway 62 at Fort Klamath onto Nicholson Road. Following signs to Sevenmile trailhead, turn right on Road 3334 and follow it 5.5 miles to the roadend.

> *Note: The Forest Service is considering relocating the Sevenmile trailhead 1.3 miles to the northeast, which would add to the length of this hike.*

The Fourmile Lake Trailhead in the south is reached by taking Road 3661 off Highway 140 across from Lake of the Woods.

INTRODUCTION South of Crater Lake the Cascade Range narrows somewhat, but packed tightly into this mountainous strip is a beautiful land of open forests, deep canyons, craggy mountains, and countless lakes. Such features long ago made the Sky Lakes Wilderness a popular destination for local outdoor lovers. Now their private hideaway is increasingly being discovered by hikers from other regions as word of this area's beauty spreads. This highly attractive end-to-end hike samples most of the charms of this wilderness and is equally scenic in either direction. It is described here from north to south so you can

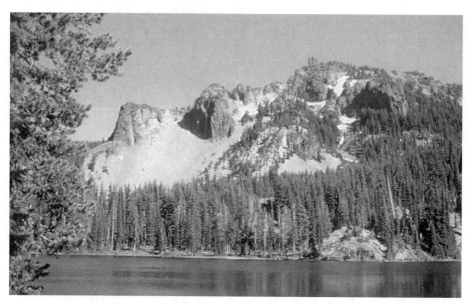

Devils Peak over Cliff Lake

enjoy a gradual approach to Mount McLoughlin, the area's principal landmark.

Warning: *The numerous lakes and ponds of the Sky Lakes Wilderness are a nursery for a tremendous population of invertebrate vampires. If you come in July—when the crags are streaked with snow and pictures are at their prettiest—be prepared with repellent, a headnet, and a well-enclosed tent. Otherwise, consider visiting from mid-August to early September, when the bugs are mostly gone and the huckleberries are ripe.*

DESCRIPTION From the Sevenmile Trailhead follow the dusty but mostly level Seven Lakes Trail past a marshy area and through a forest of lodgepole pines to a junction with the Pacific Crest Trail.

Tip: *An interesting side trip from here goes north and then west to gushing Ranger Spring—the source of the Middle Fork Rogue River.*

Continue south on the PCT for 2.5 miles to aptly named Grass Lake. A short side trail leads to a camping area on the lake's northeast shore and the first good view of craggy Devils Peak. From Grass Lake you route veers right, away from the PCT, and follows the southeast shore of the lake to a junction near Middle Lake. There are good to excellent camps at this and all the nearby lakes.

An outstanding dayhike from a base camp at any of the scenic lakes in this area turns north at Middle Lake. The path travels past North Lake on its way to tiny Lake Ivern.

Tip: A few hundred feet north of this pool is Boston Bluff and an outstanding viewpoint of the impressive glacial canyon of the Middle Fork Rogue River.

From Lake Ivern set a northwest course and walk cross-country 0.4 mile to reach a trail coming up from the Middle Fork Canyon. Turn left and follow this trail to a junction, where you turn left again and climb a ridge to narrow and remarkably straight Lake Alta, a nice place for a swim. Continue south to a junction with the western access trail for the Seven Lakes Basin and turn left. This path drops into the basin, first visiting South Lake, before arriving at Cliff Lake—most dramatic of all. Cliff Lake sits directly beneath the towering north face of Devils Peak so you should allow time to admire this spectacular spot. Excellent diving rocks are found on the far shore. To close the loop, continue north a short distance back to Middle Lake.

To continue your trip, exit the basin by heading south on the Pacific Crest Trail as it climbs the northeast shoulder of Devils Peak to a saddle beside Lee Peak.

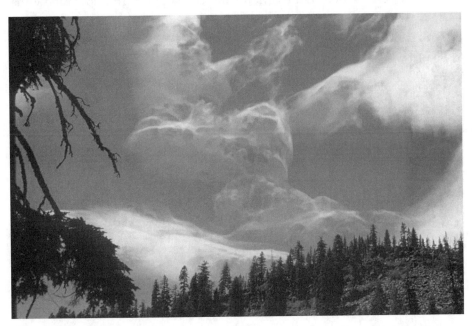

Clouds over Sky Lakes Basin

The PCT goes west across an open slope to a junction with the trail coming up from Lake Alta. Turn left and hike south along a very scenic ridge with excellent views to distant Mount McLoughlin. After 1.9 miles a trail goes northeast to nearby Upper Snow Lakes before dropping into the Sky Lakes Basin. A more scenic approach to the Sky Lakes is to continue south on the PCT for another mile and then turn left on the spectacular Divide Trail. This route descends past ponds and viewpoints to lovely Margurette Lake, where there are excellent camps.

Tip: A nice side trip from here goes north about 1.3 miles to Lower Snow Lakes, directly below the cliffs of Luther Mountain. Return via a short loop around quiet Deep and Donna lakes.

To continue your hike, go south past Trapper Lake and then through generally viewless forests for 2.1 miles to the two Heavenly Twin Lakes—largest of another attractive cluster of lakes, although these lack mountain views.

The trail crosses a narrow, forested peninsula between North and South Heavenly Twin Lakes, and then it continues southwest for 1.5 miles back to a junction with the PCT, which has made a mostly forested descent from Luther Mountain to this point. You now follow the

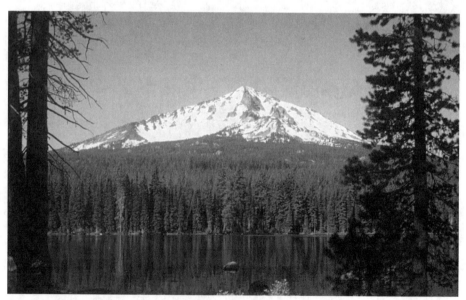

Mount McLoughlin over Squaw Lake

PCT 0.9 mile to another junction and once again turn off the main path, this time to the right on the Red Lake Trail. You pass the shores of the trail's namesake before reaching appropriately named Island Lake. In addition to a forested island, this lake has a nice view of Mount McLoughlin from a camp on its northeast shore. The path then works southeast away from the lake to a junction. Turn right and pass near the southern shore of Island Lake and an interesting historic landmark. In 1888 Judge John B. Waldo, for whom Waldo Lake was named, carved his name in a tree here during his epic exploration of the Cascade Range.

Leaving Island Lake and the "Waldo Tree" behind, go west and make a forested descent into a fifth lake basin. This one features Pear and Horseshoe lakes, both barely touched by the trail, and several off-trail pools. Prettiest, and most popular, of the lakes here is Blue Lake, backed by a 300-foot cliff. You reach this lake via a short side trip to the north at a junction west of Horseshoe Lake. There are plenty of options for campsites throughout this basin. To complete your journey, turn southwest from Blue Lake and climb 1.1 miles to a ridgetop junction. Turn left here and travel over Cat Hill, where an opening in the trees provides a nice if partly obstructed view of Mount McLoughlin.

When you yet again reach the Pacific Crest Trail, turn right (south) and gradually go up and down, mostly in forest, to a saddle with a four-way junction. Turn left and soon reach shallow Squaw Lake.

Tip: Don't miss taking a short side trip up the trailless east shore of Squaw Lake. Photographers will especially like the excellent reflection of Mount McLoughlin in the tranquil early morning waters.

The trip ends with an almost level forest walk to the south end of Fourmile "Lake" (actually a human-made reservoir).

POSSIBLE ITINERARY

	Camp	Miles	Elevation Gain
Day 1	Cliff Lake	5.2	800
Day 2	Cliff Lake (Lake Ivern dayhike loop)	9.8	1400
Day 3	Margurette Lake	11.0	1600
Day 4	Blue Lake	11.7	500
Day 5	Out	6.9	900

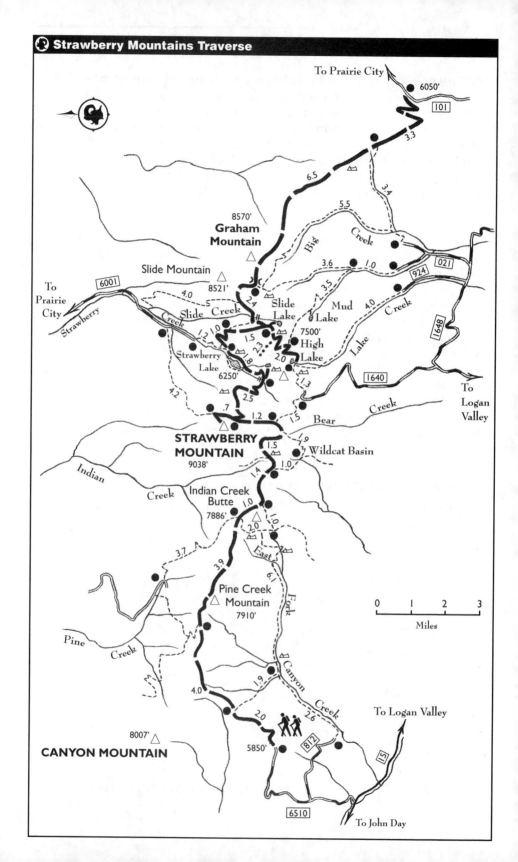

15 Strawberry Mountains Traverse

RATINGS (1–10)			MILES	ELEVATION GAIN	DAYS	SHUTTLE MILEAGE
Scenery	Solitude	Difficulty				
9	6	7	35	7600	4	31
			(52)	(11,700)	(5–6)	

MAP USFS—*Strawberry Mountain Wilderness*

USUALLY OPEN Late June to early November

BEST Early to mid-July/mid-October

PERMITS None

RULES No camping within 100 feet of lakes or streams; maximum group size of 12 people/18 stock

CONTACT Prairie City Ranger District, (541) 820-3800

SPECIAL ATTRACTIONS Mountain scenery; views; fall colors; solitude (for most of the trip); wildlife

PROBLEMS Long stretches without water; recent burn area

HOW TO GET THERE To find the west trailhead, take Highway 395 south from Canyon City for 8 miles and then turn left (east) onto paved County Road 65 (Forest Road 15) for 3 miles. Turn left on gravel Road 6510 and follow it to its end at the Joaquin Miller Trailhead. To reach the east trailhead, continue on Road 15 and then take Road 16 through Logan Valley to Summit Prairie. Turn north for 3.2 miles on Road 14 and then west on rough gravel Road 101 for 1.4 miles to the Skyline Trailhead.

> *Note: In 1996 the Wildcat Fire swept through a large section of the Strawberry Mountain Wilderness. On this hike, the affected area extends from Indian Creek Butte in the west to Twin Springs Basin on the east side of Strawberry Mountain. While flowers and grasses have benefited from the blaze, many views now include large areas of snags*

and blackened timber. Shade is at a premium on this section of the trail. In addition, trails will be plagued for several years by lots of downed snags.

INTRODUCTION The narrow spine of the Strawberry Mountains packs a lot of scenic punch in a small package. Its snowy line of peaks provides a lovely backdrop seen both from the north over the upper John Day River Valley near Prairie City and from the south over Logan Valley. Happily, the backcountry trails provide scenery at least as good as that seen from a distance. Views are spectacular throughout, flowers are abundant, and wildlife is unusually common. The range is crowded only near the few lakes in it, so there are miles of rarely traveled trails. For those who do make the scenic traverse of the Strawberries, most begin at the Canyon Mountain Trailhead near Iron King Mine. The route described here is shorter, involves less climbing, and has better road access. It also passes through some of the range's best wildlife habitat, so your chances of seeing elk, bighorn sheep, and other animals are significantly improved.

DESCRIPTION This trip starts with a short climb up Rattlesnake Ridge followed by three long downhill switchbacks to a saddle. Now you contour around two hills and then drop a bit to another saddle and a junction with the Tamarack Creek Trail where you go left.

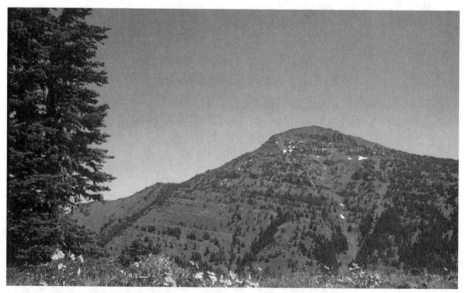

Strawberry Mountain from ridge near Indian Creek Butte

Tip: This is one of the best areas in Oregon to spot bighorn sheep. Keep your binoculars handy for the next few miles. If you're really lucky, you may also see black bears or the elusive mountain lion. Watch for movement on the steep canyon walls of Berry and Tamarack creeks.

From the junction your trail climbs steeply up a ridge and then contours around the head of Tamarack Creek.

Tip: At a saddle on the side of this ridge, be sure to visit a small rise south of the trail to check out the view and look for animals.

The climb eases somewhat as you approach a pass along the high ridge of the Strawberry Mountains. For the next several miles the route follows this view-packed ridge. Water is scarce except for a few snow patches into July.

Keep right at a junction with the Canyon Mountain Trail and then cut across the steep north face of Pine Creek Mountain. Snow lingers here for much of the season. Your trail climbs to a pass on the east slopes of Pine Creek Mountain and then makes a long traverse along the south side of the ridge. The trail remains on the south side as it makes a gradual descent to a four-way junction, immediately north of prominent Indian Creek Butte.

Tip: Camps in this area are best made either near the previous crossings of two small creeks, or by turning right and dropping 500 feet in 1.5 miles to a spring with a good campsite.

Note: From this point to a little beyond Strawberry Mountain, the 1996 Wildcat Fire made great changes to the landscape.

The main trail stays straight at the four-way junction and cuts across the east face of Indian Creek Butte. To the east, across the deep canyon of Indian Creek, rises Strawberry Mountain, the highest point in this range. The trail contours through a low saddle to a trail junction. Turn left and travel east along the ridge to a large meadow that supports scattered wildflowers in July and has an exceptionally picturesque view of Strawberry Mountain. From here the trail drops to a junction where there is a choice of trails. To the right, the main trail drops to the wildflowers of Wildcat Basin (good camps) before climbing through an interesting eroded "badlands" back up to the ridge. A shorter but equally scenic alternate route, from the junction goes left, passes a junction with the Indian Creek Trail, and soon reaches a beautiful little meadow at the head of Indian Creek. This marshy basin holds lots of wildflowers, provides a fine view of the cliffs to the south, and has good camps.

Warning: This boggy area supports a healthy mosquito population through July.

From Indian Creek you make several switchbacks up to a ridge and then reunite with the main trail climbing up from Wildcat Basin. Hike east and climb to the end of a closed jeep road that now serves as a trail. You turn left here and follow this exposed and rocky trail north, passing several exceptional vistas to the west.

At a ridgetop junction, drop your heavy pack, pick up a camera, and then head north for an excellent side trip to the summit of Strawberry Mountain. The route first cuts across the rocky east face of the peak, where you'll enjoy terrific views to the east. A short side trail climbs the northeast ridge to the top. On a clear day there seems to be no end to the views from this grandstand. To the north is the John Day River Valley. To the west is the crumpled spine of the Strawberry Range, with the Aldrich and Ochoco mountains in the distance. On very clear days even the snowy peaks of the Cascades can be seen. To the south are the forested Blue Mountains and distant Steens Mountain. Turning east you will see the scenic peaks, cliffs, and lake basins that will occupy your attention for the next couple of days. A sharp eye will even be able to spot the Elkhorn Range and part of the Wallowa Mountains to the northeast.

After absorbing the views, return to your pack and begin the long descent east toward Strawberry Lake. The highly scenic trail goes through Twin Springs Basin (good camps) and then rounds a ridge with excellent views of Strawberry Lake and the cliffs surrounding this basin. About 1,000 feet further down you reach a crossing of Strawberry Creek and a junction. To the right is a highly recommended 0.6-mile side trip to beautiful Little Strawberry Lake. The lake sits at the base of 1,500-foot cliffs, so bring an extra-wide-angle lens for photographs. There are good camps at both Little Strawberry Lake and Strawberry Creek.

Tip: These camps are generally less crowded than those farther down the trail at popular Strawberry Lake.

To continue your trip, return to the main trail and switchback down the forested slope to the north, stopping along the way to enjoy Strawberry Falls. At the south end of 31-acre Strawberry Lake is a junction. The trail along the west shore is more scenic, but the shorter route along the east side is the usual choice.

Tip: At the north end be sure to take a short detour along the lake's northwest shore to enjoy a classic view across the lake of the jagged snowy ridge above. Afternoons provide the best lighting for photographs. Since the lake's water level fluctuates considerably, early summer is best.

Camps (and people) are abundant near Strawberry Lake, so if you camp here, expect plenty of company and heed all Forest Service restrictions on where to set up your tent.

Keep right at two junctions not far below the lake's outlet, following signs to Slide Lake. The trail climbs steadily to a junction at a flat spot on the ridge. The quickest exit goes left, but taking it would miss too much great scenery, so keep right and make a long up-and-down traverse across an open slope. The distinctive peak to the east is Slide Mountain. Reenter woods and keep right at a junction before climbing to a second junction. To the left is the short side trail to scenic Slide Lake, which has excellent camps.

Slide Lake makes an outstanding base camp for dayhikes. Possible hikes range from the short stroll to Little Slide Lake, a small pool about 0.2 mile south of Slide Lake, to the long scramble up Slide Mountain. Probably the two most spectacular destinations can be combined in one rugged day. Begin by climbing the trail heading southwest from the Slide Lake junction. Leave the trail near the base of a steep talus slope and scramble up the ridge to the northwest. The climb ends at the top of the high cliffs above Little Strawberry Lake. If you're not afraid of heights, this is a grand spot to dangle your legs over the edge of a precipice and enjoy the view.

To continue your dayhike excursion, return to the trail, turn right, and climb across a steep, rocky slope to a pass.

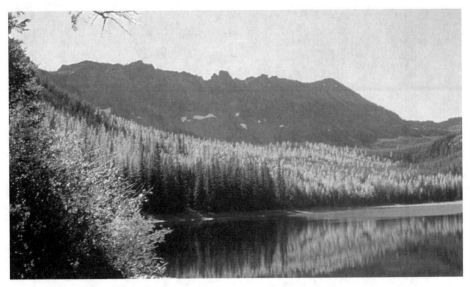

Strawberry Lake

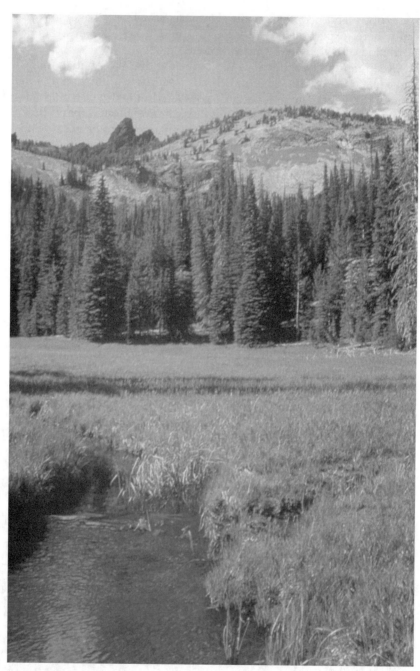

Meadow below High Lake

Warning: *This slope is usually covered with steep snowfields until about mid-July.*

Keep right at a junction and travel along the top of an open ridge, where windswept trees and small alpine wildflowers enhance the wonderful scenery. The path now makes a long descent to High Lake—a spectacular pool backed by high cliffs and ridges. Once you've had your fill, return to Slide Lake the way you came.

To complete your tour, return to the junction north of Slide Lake and turn right. As the trail drops to a junction, look for fine views up to Slide Mountain. Turn right and continue downhill to a creek crossing.

Tip: *Impressive Slide Falls is a short bushwhack upstream.*

The trail now makes a long 1,200-foot climb out of Slide Basin. Along the way you turn right at a junction with the newly constructed Slide Basin Connector Trail and then complete your climb to a pass with another trail junction. South of the pass is Big Riner Basin (good campsites) and to the left is Graham Mountain.

Turn left at the junction, staying on the Skyline Trail as it makes a long traverse across the southwest slopes of Graham Mountain. You reach a saddle and begin following a scenic up-and-down ridge. To the east, across the forested upper John Day River Valley, are Lookout and Glacier mountains. As the route loops south around Dead Horse Basin it stays on the west side of the ridge and passes two welcome springs. Views to the west are superb.

The trail returns to the increasingly forested ridgecrest and eventually meets the Snowshoe Trail coming up from a recently fire-scarred area to the west. The Skyline Trail continues straight, staying along the ridge for another mile before dropping in very long switchbacks to the eastern trailhead on Road 101.

POSSIBLE ITINERARY			
	Camp	Miles	Elevation Gain
Day 1	Spring below Indian Creek Butte	11.4	3000
Day 2	Twin Springs Basin (with side trip up Strawberry Mountain)	9.6	3100
Day 3	Slide Lake (with side trip to Little Strawberry Lake)	7.3	1300
Day 4	Slide Lake (dayhike to High Lake and Strawberry Ridge)	11.0	2400
Day 5	Out	12.5	1900

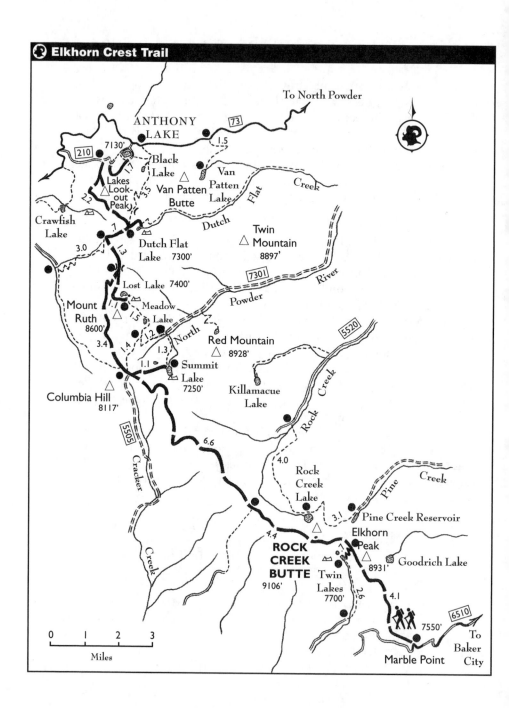

To North Powder

ANTHONY LAKE
73
7130'
1.5
210
1.7
Black Lake
Van Patten Lake
Van Patten Butte
Lakes Look-out Peak
3.5
2.2
Crawfish Lake
.7
1.3
Dutch Flat Lake 7300'
Dutch Flat
Creek
Twin Mountain 8897'
3.0
7301
Lost Lake 7400'
Powder
River
Mount Ruth 8600'
1.1
Meadow Lake
1.5
1.5
5520
3.4
1.4
1.2
North
Red Mountain 8928'
1.3
1.1
Summit Lake 7250'
Columbia Hill 8117'
Killamacue Lake
Rock
Creek
5505
6.6
Cracker
4.0
Rock Creek Lake
Pine
Creek
Creek
3.1
Pine Creek Reservoir
4.4
Elkhorn Peak
ROCK CREEK BUTTE 9106'
.7
8931'
Goodrich Lake
Twin Lakes 7700'
2.6
4.1
6510
7550'
To Baker City
Marble Point

0   1   2   3
Miles

16 Elkhorn Crest Trail

RATINGS (1–10)			MILES	ELEVATION GAIN	DAYS	SHUTTLE MILEAGE
Scenery	Solitude	Difficulty				
9	6	6	28	3000	3	33
			(33)	(5700)	(3–4)	

MAP USGS—*Elkhorn Peak, Bourne, and Anthony Lakes*

USUALLY OPEN July to October

BEST Mid-July

PERMITS None

RULES The Forest Service *recommends* a maximum group size of 12 people/18 stock and camping at least 100 feet from lakes and streams

CONTACT Whitman Ranger District, (541) 523-4476

SPECIAL ATTRACTIONS Views; granite peaks, cirque lakes, and generally excellent mountain scenery; relative solitude

PROBLEMS Poor road access to southern trailhead; motorbikes

HOW TO GET THERE To reach the north trailhead at Anthony Lake, take Interstate 84 to the North Powder exit. Turn west and follow signs to Anthony Lakes as you climb paved Road 73 to the Anthony Lake Campground.

Tip: The best place to park is a bit east of the campground at the well-marked Elkhorn Crest Trailhead.

The south trailhead is more difficult to reach. From Highway 30 just north of Baker City, turn west on Pocahontas Road and follow it for 6.5 miles to the third sharp right turn. Turn left onto Road 6510 which enters national forest land and passes the Marble Creek Picnic Area.

Warning: The road surface gets rougher as you continue to climb. High-clearance vehicles are recommended.

You pass through a gravel quarry and eventually top out at a pass and the Marble Point Trailhead.

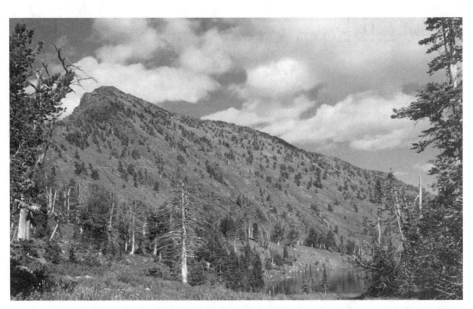

Elkhorn Peak over Lower Twin Lake

INTRODUCTION The jagged spine of the Elkhorn Range rises dramatically above Baker City and the Powder River Valley. Strangely, although countless thousands of people drive past these impressive peaks on Interstate 84, relatively few stop to explore. This narrow range hides many of the same treasures that make the nearby Wallowa Mountains so popular (granite peaks, glacial lakes, and clear streams), but for some reason it receives only a tiny fraction of the publicity. Lovers of solitude would prefer it stayed that way. Unfortunately, most of this range is unprotected and therefore open to mining (once an important business in these mountains), logging, and motorbikes. A trip along the view-packed Elkhorn Crest Trail is the ideal way for backpackers to enjoy this lovely range and learn what is at stake. This relatively easy trail closely follows a high ridge for its entire length. Side trails drop to numerous lakes and meadows with scenic campsites. The trip is beautiful in either direction, but south to north is marginally easier, since the start is some 400 feet higher.

> *Warning: Sadly, the southern half of this trail is open to motorbikes. Be prepared to have the quiet disrupted on occasion.*

DESCRIPTION Your route climbs gradually up a mostly open ridge to the northwest. Views here, as is true along most of this route, are superb as they alternate between the forested Blue Mountains and Sumpter Valley to the southwest, and the Powder River Valley and the distant Wallowa Mountains to the northeast. For most of the trip the trail stays on the west side of the Elkhorn Crest, so views west dominate.

Round a bend after about one mile and begin to travel in a more northerly direction. There are outstanding views along this stretch of trail, particularly of the scenic basin holding the Twin Lakes, with brown and reddish peaks all around. The high point on the east side of this basin is Elkhorn Peak—an inviting mountain with reasonably easy access up its south ridge. The crest trail (inaccurately shown on USGS maps) continues its scenic course—sometimes on the ridge's west side, sometimes at or near the crest—for another 3 miles to a trail junction in a saddle. Don't miss the excellent side trip that turns left and drops 0.7 mile in a series of long switchbacks to Lower Twin Lake—backed by rugged cliffs. Smaller Upper Twin Lake is also worth exploring, although there is no official trail. The lower lake is more scenic and has better camps.

Fill your water bottles (there is precious little of the stuff along the ridge), climb back up to the crest trail, turn left, and round the head of the Twin Lakes Basin.

Tip: An outstanding cross-country side trip climbs moderately steep slopes to the summit of Rock Creek Butte. At 9,106 feet this is the highest point in the range, and it commands a breathtaking view in all directions. Most impressive of all is the look down to sparkling Rock Creek

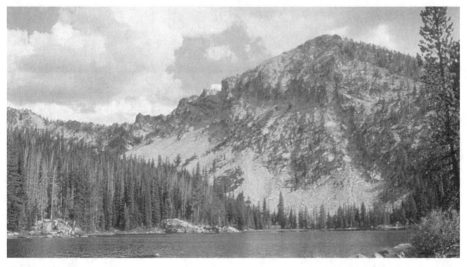

Summit Lake

Lake, sitting in a stark basin beneath sheer cliffs. Bring binoculars to check for small moving snowfields that are actually mountain goats.

After another 0.7 mile on the crest trail, scramble up to a second cliff-edge viewpoint, this time of tiny Bucket Lake. Mountain goats are common here as well.

The delightful and gently graded trail passes a junction with a rarely used path from the west and then continues for another 6.6 joyous miles of open ridges and views. Notice how the rock changes from reddish volcanic rocks to predominately white granite. The soils also become more suitable for forests and the trees grow thicker and healthier than in the sparsely vegetated Twin Lakes Basin. The only blemish on the scene is the remains of mining activity along Cracker Creek. In a saddle about 0.5 mile northeast of prominent Columbia Hill is a trail junction. From here a worthwhile side trip goes east to popular Summit Lake. This is a large, beautiful lake with good fishing, several excellent campsites, and photogenic granite cliffs above its southwest shore.

From the Summit Lake junction go west and quickly reach a four-way junction with a jeep track (still in use), where you go straight and soon reach a pass beside Columbia Hill. Your route goes north, sticking to the Elkhorn Crest Trail (#1611). The trail gradually climbs toward Mount Ruth and soon enters the North Fork John Day Wilderness, so the motorbikes are finally left behind.

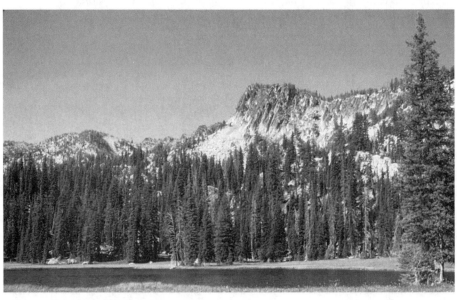

Dutch Flat Lake

Tip: The summit view from Mount Ruth amply rewards the scrambler.

The trail skirts the west side of this peak before dropping first to Lost Lake Saddle and then Nip and Tuck Pass and a junction. A highly recommended side trip drops southeast from this junction across a rocky slope and then loops around the basin holding Lost Lake (one of at least 14 lakes in Oregon holding this unimaginative name). An easy walk through open woods and meadows leads to the lake's southeast shore with views back up to Mount Ruth. Several good camps are located around this lake.

Back at Nip and Tuck Pass the crest trail continues to Cunningham Saddle and a junction with a path coming up from the west. To the north are terrific views of spacious Crawfish Meadows backed by a jagged ridge. Now you cross a slope, with intermittent views of this spectacular basin, to a pass and a junction. To the right a recommended side trail drops 600 feet to small but scenic Dutch Flat Lake, with good views and nice camps. From the pass, the official Elkhorn Crest Trail climbs north to a saddle beside Angell Peak, then drops past Black Lake on its way to the trailhead on Road 73. This scenic route is the quickest way out for those in a hurry. There is another alternative, however, that allows you to savor still more of this country. Turn left and drop about 400 feet before contouring across the slope on the north side of Crawfish Basin. You round another ridge and then climb to a junction with the 0.7-mile trail to the top of Lakes Lookout Peak. This peak provides a particularly good perspective of the Anthony Lakes area, so the side trip is well worthwhile. A short distance farther north is the end of Road 210 coming up from the west, and the top of several ski lifts for the Anthony Lakes ski area.

Keep right and descend on a road/trail that makes a long switchback. At the second switchback, keep straight on a trail leading to the small but very scenic Hoffer Lakes. Finally, drop steeply to busy Anthony Lake with its mountain views, campground, and, of course, your waiting vehicle.

POSSIBLE ITINERARY			
	Camp	Miles	Elevation Gain
Day 1	Lower Twin Lake	4.8	800
Day 2	Summit Lake	12.8	1300
Day 3	Dutch Flat Lake (with side trip to Lost Lake)	9.8	1800
Day 4	Out (with side trip to Lakes Lookout Peak)	6.1	1800

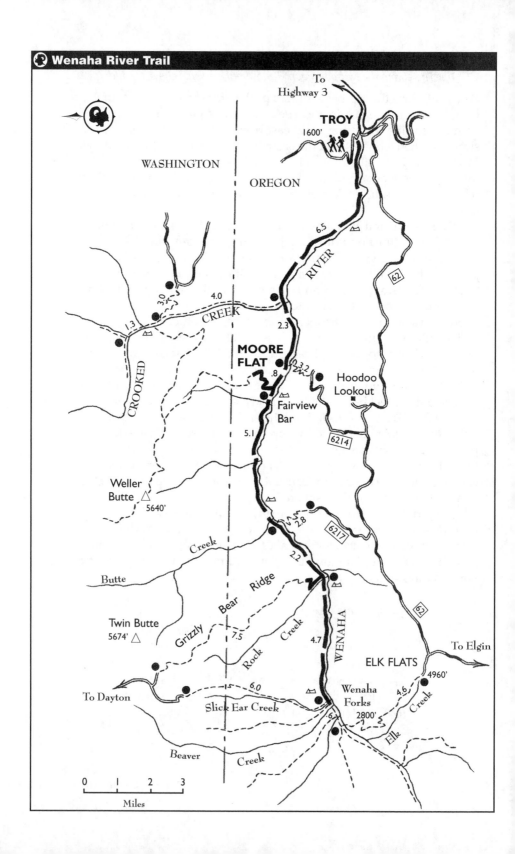

Wenaha River Trail

To
Highway 3

TROY
1600'

WASHINGTON

OREGON

6.5

RIVER

62

3.0

4.0

CREEK

1.3

2.3

CROOKED

**MOORE
FLAT**

3.2

.8

Hoodoo
Lookout

Fairview
Bar

6214

5.1

Weller
Butte
5640'

2.8

6217

Creek

2.2

Butte

Grizzly

Bear

Ridge

WENAHA

62

Twin Butte
5674'

7.5

Rock

Creek

4.7

ELK FLATS

4960'

To Elgin

To Dayton

6.0

Wenaha
Forks
2800'

4.6

Creek

Slick Ear Creek

Elk

Beaver

Creek

0   1   2   3

Miles

17 Wenaha River Trail

RATINGS (1–10)			MILES	ELEVATION GAIN	DAYS	SHUTTLE MILEAGE
Scenery	Solitude	Difficulty				
9	6	5	32	2800	3–4	22
			(49)	(4500)	(4–6)	N/A

MAP USFS—*Wenaha-Tucannon Wilderness*

USUALLY OPEN April to November

BEST May/October

PERMITS None

RULES Camp at least 75 feet from water

CONTACT Pomeroy Ranger District, (509) 843-1891

SPECIAL ATTRACTIONS Fine canyon scenery; fishing; good early-season hike; fall colors; wildlife

PROBLEMS Rattlesnakes; difficult early-season access to upper trailhead; some poison ivy

HOW TO GET THERE To reach the tiny community of Troy, drive north from Enterprise on Highway 3 for 33 miles. Turn left on the signed road to Flora and Troy. The road goes through farmland and the dilapidated buildings in Flora and then turns to gravel as it winds steeply down into the Grande Ronde River Canyon. Cross the bridge, drive to the north end of town, and then turn west on the gravel road to Pomeroy. You will reach the marked trailhead at a switchback in the road just 0.3 mile from town. If it's not snowed in, the upstream trailhead at Elk Flats is reached by driving west on Forest Road 62, which begins off the Grande Ronde River Road about 0.5 mile south of Troy. After 20 miles turn right for 0.7 mile to the signed trailhead.

INTRODUCTION For countless thousands of years, the Wenaha River has been carving a canyon into the lava tablelands of Oregon's Blue Mountains. The result of these relentless efforts is a spectacular 2,000-foot-deep chasm. The scenic mix includes a clear rushing stream, open ponderosa-pine forests, steep grasslands covered with wildflowers,

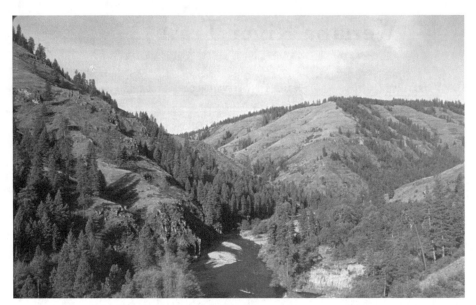

Wenaha River Canyon below Crooked Creek

and rugged rock outcroppings. The best way to appreciate the river's handiwork is to hike the full length of the Wenaha River Trail—one of Oregon's classic wild-river and canyon tours.

Although it's only a short distance from much better-known Hells Canyon, the Wenaha River Canyon differs considerably in character. From a strictly practical standpoint the Wenaha Canyon has the advantage, since it has better road access and an easier trail. Also, while rattlesnakes are found in both places, poison ivy, a continuous menace in Hells Canyon, is found only in the lower Wenaha Canyon and is easily avoided. From a scenery standpoint, Hells Canyon has the edge, due to its greater depth and continuous jaw-dropping views. But the Wenaha River's scenery is still great and will impress even the most well-traveled hiker. Probably the most noticeable difference—especially on a hot day in late spring or summer—is that this canyon has trees. Beautiful old ponderosa pines are welcome companions throughout the hike, and these are often joined by cottonwood, Douglas fir, and grand fir. The trees sometimes block the view, but their welcome shade is a real blessing.

DESCRIPTION With the cooperation of Mother Nature this would be an easy, point to point, downhill hike. Unfortunately, in the spring (when the lower canyon is at its best) the upper trailhead is typically snowed in. One solution is to do this trip in October when the sumac bushes and maples turn color and temperatures have cooled. The other alternative—described here—is an up-and-back hike in the spring from the lower trailhead at Troy.

If the upper trailhead is open, hike downstream from Elk Flats to Troy—a trip that involves almost no elevation gain. For an upstream trip from Troy, begin by gradually dropping to the first of several grassy river-level flats. This one features a row of pungent lilac bushes. The trail alternates between river-level flats and grassy slopes and benches with scattered ponderosa pines. The canyon slopes consist of open grasslands and rocky ledges with lots of colorful spring wildflowers. Excellent views along this stretch are too numerous to list and possible side trips to the clear stream are frequent and highly rewarding. As the trail goes up the canyon, the pines gradually become more numerous and wetter sections support thickets of bushes and tall grasses. The canyon walls also get steeper and rockier.

Tip: *Keep a sharp eye on the ledges above the trail for bighorn sheep—common in this area.*

Pass through a gate at 4.5 miles and enter the wilderness at 6.0 miles. At 6.5 miles is a trail junction and the bridged crossing of Crooked Creek. Be alert for white-tailed deer (found in only a few parts of Oregon), as well as coyote, porcupine, rattlesnake, and a wide variety of birds.

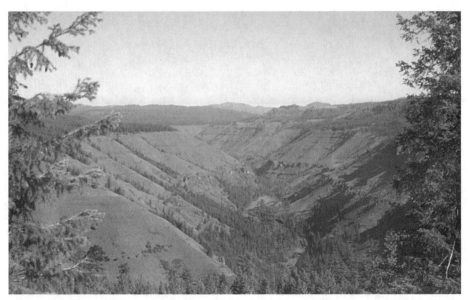

Wenaha River Canyon near Troy

In another 2 miles is a junction with the Hoodoo Trail, which has no bridge to accommodate its crossing of the river. The ford is easy in the fall, but too dangerous for most hikers in the spring. If you can cross, the trail that switchbacks up the opposite canyon wall is well worth a side trip.

The main Wenaha River Trail continues its very scenic tour upriver to Fairview Bar—a large, grassy flat with ponderosa pines and good camps. From Fairview Bar a poorly marked but not-to-be-missed side trail goes north to Moore Flat. The path is initially overgrown and hard to find, but soon it becomes a good trail as it climbs the hillside. About 1.5 miles up this sometimes steep trail is a huge, dry, grassy slope. Flowers here include phlox, lupine, balsamroot, and clarkia, and the views up the canyon are outstanding.

Five scenic miles upstream from Fairview Bar is the junction with the Cross Canyon Trail, which has dropped to the river from a trailhead on the south rim. Energetic hikers might want to take a side trip up this steep, view-packed trail. The main river trail continues to fair camps near Rock Creek and a junction.

An outstanding side trip turns right at Rock Creek. The route closely follows the stream for about 0.7 mile and then turns away from the brushy creek and climbs to a switchback on Grizzly Bear Ridge. From here there is a particularly photogenic view downstream with fir trees

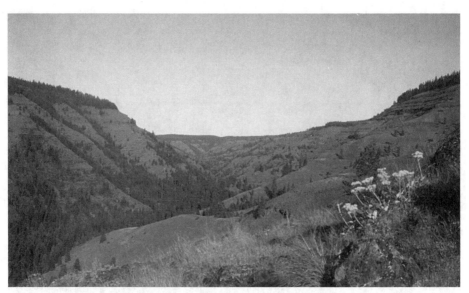

Wenaha Canyon from near Moore Flat

to frame the scene. This is a great place to spend some time enjoying the river's handiwork.

This side trip is a logical turnaround point, but there is more good canyon scenery ahead. The trend of gradually thicker forests and a wetter environment continues as you go upriver for 4.7 miles to the Wenaha Forks, where several canyons and their braided streams converge. In this area Slick Ear Creek, Beaver Creek, and the north and south forks of the Wenaha River all come together to form the main stream. Beavers work these waters and other wildlife is abundant. Good camps can be found in several places.

Wenaha Forks is the best turnaround point, as the canyon trail from here follows the much smaller South Fork and views become increasingly restricted. Several other paths radiate up the various creeks and ridges that converge here. To reach the Elk Flats Trailhead, cross the South Fork Wenaha River and climb a moderately graded trail through cool forests for 4.6 miles to the trailhead. Canyon views are limited and rather disappointing on this path.

POSSIBLE ITINERARY

	Camp	Miles	Elevation Gain
Day 1	Fairview Bar	9.6	500
Day 2	Rock Creek (with side trip to Moore Flat)	10.3	2200
Day 3	Rock Creek (dayhike to Wenaha Forks and Grizzly Bear Ridge)	11.8	1500
Day 4	Crooked Creek	10.4	200
Day 5	Out	6.5	100

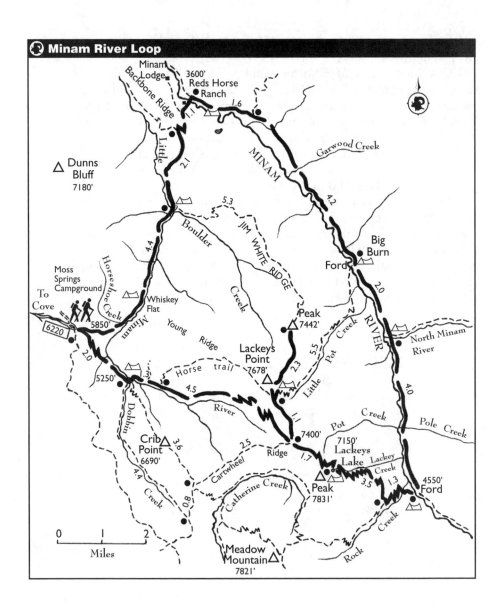

Minam
Lodge

Backbone Ridge

3600'
Reds Horse
Ranch

1.6

1.1

Dunns
Bluff
7180'

Little

2.1

Garwood Creek

MINAM

4.2

5.3

Boulder

JIM WHITE RIDGE

Big
Burn

Ford

Creek

2.0

Moss
Springs
Campground

Horseshoe Creek

To
Cove

6220

5850'

Whiskey
Flat

Young

Ridge

Peak
7442'

RIVER

North Minam
River

Minam

Lackeys
Point
7678'

5.5

Little

Pot

Creek

2.3

5250'

1.3

Horse

trail

4.5

River

4.0

7400'

1.1

Pot

Creek

Pole Creek

Crib
Point
6690'

3.6

Dobbin

2.5

Ridge

1.7

7150'
Lackeys
Lake

Lackey
Creek

4.4

Cartwheel

Creek

0.8

Catherine Creek

Peak
7831'

3.5

1.3

4550'
Ford

0   1   2

Miles

Meadow
Mountain
7821'

Rock

Creek

18 Minam River Loop

RATINGS (1–10)			MILES	ELEVATION GAIN	DAYS	SHUTTLE MILEAGE
Scenery	Solitude	Difficulty				
7	6	7	35	5300	3–6	N/A
			(41)	(5900)	(4–6)	

MAP Imus Geographics—*Wallowa Mountains*

USUALLY OPEN July to October

BEST July

PERMIT Yes (free at the trailhead)

RULES Maximum group size of 12 people

CONTACT Wallowa Valley visitor center, (541) 426-4978

SPECIAL ATTRACTIONS Diverse scenery, including deep canyons, high ridges, and fine viewpoints; solitude

PROBLEMS Confusing junctions with unmapped trails; faint trails; heavy horse use

HOW TO GET THERE From La Grande, take exit 261 off Interstate 84, and drive 1.5 miles northeast on State Highway 82 to a major junction. Go straight (east) on State Highway 237 and proceed 13.8 miles to Cove. One block after the road makes a 90-degree turn to the right (west), turn left (south) on French Street, which soon becomes Mill Creek Lane. Remain on this road, which turns to gravel after 2.1 miles and becomes Forest Road 6220, and drive 9.1 miles to the trailhead at the east end of horse-oriented Moss Springs Campground.

INTRODUCTION Although this western third of the Eagle Cap Wilderness is easier for most Oregonians to reach, who drive from the populous Willamette Valley, it receives far fewer visitors than the central portion of the preserve. The reason for this seeming incongruity is that this part of the wilderness has none of the fish-filled lakes or high granite peaks that draw crowds to other parts of the Wallowa Mountains. Nonetheless, there is still plenty of great scenery, most notably high alpine ridges that boast terrific views, plenty of wildflowers, and the

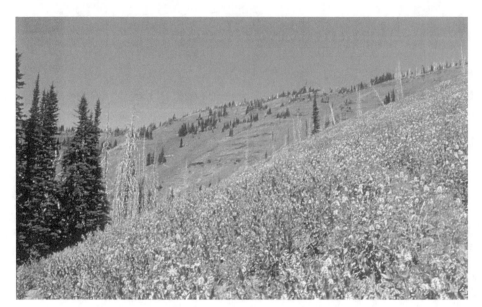

Flowers along Little Minam Trail, Jim White Ridge

remarkably clear Minam River, which flows through an impressive 3500-foot-deep forested canyon. In addition, while you probably won't have the trails all to yourself, you also won't have to fight off other backpackers for a good campsite, which is sometimes a problem in the more popular areas to the east.

DESCRIPTION Start by walking east from the trailhead and soon pick up a dusty, horse-pounded trail that goes through a pleasant forest of western larches, mountain hemlocks, Engelmann spruces, lodgepole pines, and subalpine firs. After only 70 yards, the trail splits at the start of the loop.

A counterclockwise tour is preferable because it avoids a long climb out of the Minam River Canyon, so bear right, following signs to Upper Little Minam. For 1.5 miles you gradually lose elevation in four lazy switchbacks to the bottom of the canyon of the Little Minam River. Here you hop over a tiny creek and then walk 0.5 mile through an open lodgepole-pine forest to a junction with the Art Garrett Trail. Go straight and, 100 yards later, make a log crossing of clear Dobbin Creek. Just 50 yards later is a nice campsite and another junction, this time with Crib Point Trail. Veer left and immediately cross the gravel-strewn Little Minam River on a log.

The trail now goes upstream, gradually gaining elevation through a mix of forest and small meadows. In early July these meadows are filled with tall wildflowers, including false hellebore, mariposa lily, horsemint, sunflower, pink geranium, and bluebells. About 0.8 mile from the crossing of the Little Minam River, go straight at a confusing and unmapped junction with an unofficial horse trail that goes uphill to the left. Just 0.5 mile farther, go straight again at a junction with another unmapped equestrian trail, this one an unofficial shortcut to Jim White Ridge.

> **Warning:** *These are only the first of many unofficial horse trails that you will encounter on this trip. Confusingly, many of these paths appear to get more use than the official Forest Service trails. Keep your map handy and consult it often to ensure that you are headed in the proper direction.*

After these junctions, the trail gradually pulls away from the river (now just a creek), ascending at a steady but moderate grade on a partly forested hillside. Several tiny side creeks provide water on this long 2200-foot climb. About one-third of the way up you enter the Little Minam Burn, a decades-old blaze that left many snags but opened up fine views of the high ridges flanking this canyon. The most interesting of these ridges lies straight ahead to the southeast, tempting the hiker with its open, rounded slopes that promise fine views. This enticing ridge is your goal, but it is still a long way up, so settle in for a lengthy trudge. A total of six switchbacks add variety along the way, but it is the increasingly excellent scenery that really keeps you going. Views of the nearby ridges and the distant Grande Ronde Valley and Elkhorn and Blue mountains are more impressive with each upward step. In July, wildflowers compete with the views for your attention. Expect colorful displays of Sitka valerian, paintbrush, buckwheat, lupine, and scarlet gilia. The large sloping meadows here seem even more expansive because many of the trees were burned in the Little Minam Fire. At 7.8 miles from the trailhead, you reach a four-way junction marked by a prominent post just below the top of Cartwheel Ridge.

Here you have a choice. The recommended longer trail goes straight, heading for Lackeys Lake and the Minam River. If you prefer a shorter, 21-mile loop that skips the Minam River, you can take the Jim White Ridge Trail to the left. Even if you are taking the longer loop, however, you will want to take a day to explore the first few miles of Jim White Ridge because this area features terrific wildflower displays and outstanding views. So turn left (north) and ramble up and down through rolling alpine meadows that feature the usual assortment of high-elevation flora and fauna. Of the latter, look for elk lounging in the meadows, coyotes trotting by in search of ground squirrels, and mountain bluebirds and Clark's nutcrackers flying overhead. Plantlife here includes pink heather, whitebark pines, and numerous grasses and small wildflowers. At 1.1 miles from the four-way junction there is a signed junction with the Little Pot Creek Trail.

Tip: Just 0.1 mile down the Little Pot Creek Trail is an excellent campsite on a scenic little bench beside a small spring. This is a good spot to use as a base camp for exploring Jim White Ridge.

Warning: If you look at the map, the Little Pot Creek Trail appears to be a good shortcut to the Minam River. This route, however, is often sketchy and involves a tricky ford of the river at the end. The longer trail via Lackeys Lake, described below, is a much better option.

About 100 yards past the Little Pot Creek junction, the Jim White Ridge Trail comes to a fork at a cairn. The unofficial horse trail to the left is the route mentioned earlier that drops to the Little Minam River Trail at the unsigned junction 1.3 miles from the crossing of that stream. The less obvious and lesser used official trail goes right (uphill) from the cairn. This sketchy but wildly scenic path soon climbs to nearly the top of 7678-foot Lackeys Point and then drops briefly but steeply on a rocky trail (not recommended for livestock) before going up and down along the ridge to the north. There are acres of flowers here in July and terrific views in all directions. You can hike for several miles, but a logical turnaround point is a high viewpoint about 2 miles past Lackeys Point.

Returning to the four-way junction on Cartwheel Ridge, those taking the recommended loop should go southeast and, 0.1 mile later, top the rounded ridge at a point featuring fine views southwest down to the forests and meadows beside Catherine Creek, some 2000 feet below. The often narrow but mostly level trail then cuts across the steep slopes on the southwest side of a ridge for 0.7 mile before crossing over to the northeastern side of this ridge. Here views shift to the high snowy peaks of the central Wallowa Mountains towering above the deep chasm of Minam River Canyon. From here four downhill switchbacks and a gently descending traverse of a mostly wooded slope take you down to a small saddle over a spur ridge. You then drop briefly in one switchback to a crossing of Lackey Creek just below marshy and hard-to-see Lackeys Lake. There are nice camps above the east side of this pretty little lake, but the water is too shallow for fish.

From the lake the trail goes steadily downhill, losing 2600 feet on its way to the bottom of the Minam River Canyon. Fortunately, the route is well graded, but anyone taking this loop in the opposite direction will find the climb very tiring. Initially the descent is through a sloping meadow immediately below the lake. Then the trail crosses Lackey Creek a couple of times and enters forest. A dozen switchbacks over the next 3.5

miles take you to an unsigned junction with the lightly used trail to Meadow Mountain and North Catherine Creek. Go left (downhill) and make 19 short switchbacks in 1.1 miles to an aging wooden bridge over Rock Creek. Another 0.2 mile of downhill leads to a small meadow with an inviting campsite just before a ford of the crystal-clear Minam River. The water here is usually over knee-deep and quite cold, but the ford is not dangerous. Just 75 yards after the ford is a junction with the Minam River Trail.

Turn left and walk downstream on a trail that includes some minor uphills, but which is generally a long, gradual descent that never strays far from the winding Minam River. The forest and shrubbery near the water is surprisingly lush and includes ponderosa pines, Pacific yews, and thimbleberries, all species that prefer these lower elevations to the high ridges. After crossing Pole Creek on a log, you continue descending, mostly in forest, but with many lovely views of the river with high ridges rising in the background. At 4 miles from where you started on the Minam River Trail is a good camp below the trail, just before a sturdy wooden bridge over North Minam River. About 100 yards later is a junction with the North Minam River Trail, where you go straight.

About 2 miles past the North Minam junction you come to a lovely meadow named, for no obvious reason, Big Burn, with nice camps and a cairn marking the junction with the Little Pot Creek Trail. The

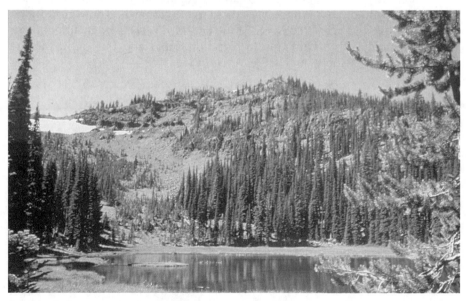

Lackeys Lake

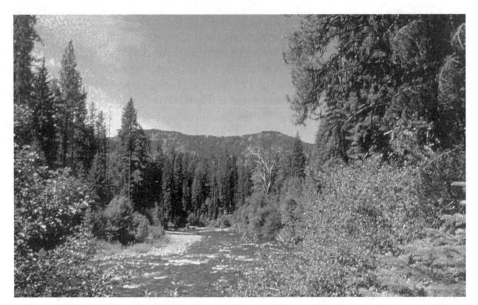

Minam River above Reds Horse Ranch

tread of this side trail is so faint it is hard to locate. Go straight and for the next 4.2 miles spend most of your time well away from the river and, illogically, seeming to go uphill. The forest scenery is rather mundane, although it is more varied as large cottonwoods now grow in the bottomlands near the river. At the end of this section, go straight at a junction with a faint trail to Standley Cabin and then return to the banks of the now quite large Minam River.

> **Tip:** *There are a couple of very nice, secluded camps along the river here, which you can reach via unsigned use paths that drop down to the left.*

About 1.6 miles from the Standley Cabin junction is a junction with Horse Ranch Trail. Turn left, immediately cross an elaborately large wooden bridge over the river, and then climb briefly to the huge meadow holding the buildings, fences, and corrals of historic Reds Horse Ranch (now run by the Forest Service). The trail goes through a gate (cleverly latched in place with horseshoes) and then across a large pasture, part of which is mowed and used as a wilderness airstrip.

> **Note:** *Be sure to close all gates behind you to keep the horses from straying.*

At the west end of the meadow, or pasture, you go through another gate and immediately come to a junction with a spur trail to privately owned Minam Lodge. This rustic but very comfortable facility offers cabin accommodations, hearty homemade meals, and a variety of outdoor-oriented activities. If you are interested in staying here as part of your trip, contact the lodge at (541) 432-6545 or www.minam-lodgeoutfitters.com.

After the Minam Lodge junction, you return to the forest, some of which has been partially burned, and begin a 700-foot climb to the top of narrow Backbone Ridge. Most of this climb is a long traverse, although there are two switchbacks as you approach the top. Just 0.1 mile past the top of the ridge is a junction with the Little Minam River Trail, which goes downhill and sharply to the right. You go straight and continue uphill, now on the west side of the ridge, before finally leveling off and then contouring until you meet up with the Little Minam River. About 2.1 miles from the last junction is a spacious but horsey campsite at the junction with the Jim White Ridge Trail. This is where you rejoin the main route if you took the shorter, 21-mile loop mentioned earlier.

Go right at the junction, crossing the Little Minam on a wooden bridge, and then follow that sparkling river upstream. This clear, rushing stream is a haven for dippers, chunky little gray birds that live along mountain streams and sing all year long. About 2.2 miles after the bridge is an excellent campsite on your left at a place called Whiskey Flat. From here, you follow the river another 0.7 mile before crossing Horseshoe Creek on a bridge and then climbing away from the water across open, sunny slopes with blooming snowberry bushes in July and nice views up the Little Minam River's canyon. After 1.5 miles of climbing, you return to the Moss Springs Trailhead and your car.

POSSIBLE ITINERARY			
	Camp	Miles	Elevation Gain
Day 1	Little Pot Creek Camp	8.9	2400
Day 2	Minam River (after dayhike out Jim White Ridge)	12.3	900
Day 3	Minam River before Reds Horse Ranch	11.2	200
Day 4	Out	8.2	2400

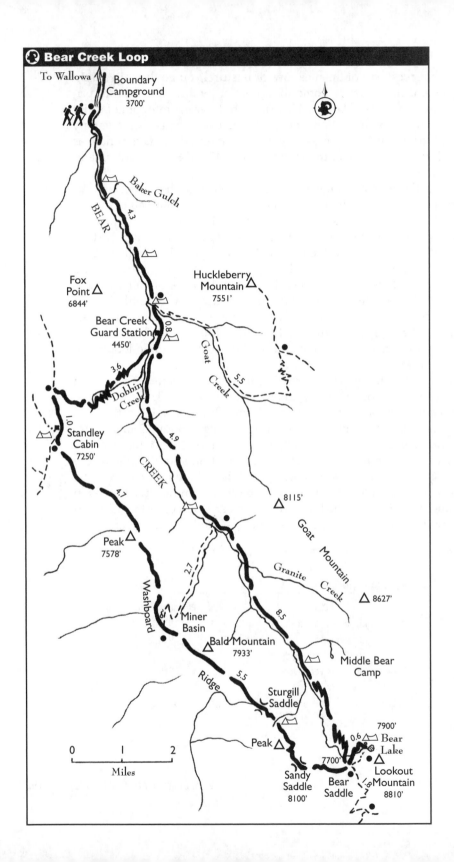

Bear Creek Loop

To Wallowa

Boundary
Campground
3700'

Baker Gulch

BEAR

4.3

Fox
Point
6844'

Huckleberry
Mountain
7551'

Bear Creek
Guard Station
4450'

0.8

Goat Creek

5.5

3.6

Dobbin
Creek

Standley
Cabin
7250'

1.0

4.9

CREEK

8115'

4.7

Goat Mountain

Peak
7578'

2.7

Granite Creek

8627'

Washboard

Miner
Basin

8.5

Bald Mountain
7933'

Middle Bear
Camp

Ridge

5.5

Sturgill
Saddle

7900'

0.6

Bear
Lake

Peak

7700'

Lookout
Mountain
8810'

Sandy
Saddle
8100'

Bear
Saddle

0

1

2

Miles

19 Bear Creek Loop

RATINGS (1–10)			MILES	ELEVATION GAIN	DAYS	SHUTTLE MILEAGE
Scenery	Solitude	Difficulty				
8	8	8	39	6300	3–6	N/A
			(40)	(6800)	4–6)	

MAP Imus Geographics—*Wallowa Mountains*

USUALLY OPEN July to October

BEST Mid-July

PERMIT Yes (free at the trailhead)

RULES Maximum group size of 12 people

CONTACT Wallowa Valley visitor center, (541) 426-4978

SPECIAL ATTRACTIONS Spectacular alpine ridge; wildlife; solitude

PROBLEMS Faint trail that often disappears; rugged hiking

HOW TO GET THERE From La Grande, take exit 261 off Interstate 84 and then drive 46 miles east on State Highway 82 to the town of Wallowa. Turn right, following signs for Boundary Campground, drive 0.3 mile, and then turn left on Bear Creek Road. Follow this paved then good gravel road for 8.1 miles to the trailhead at the south end of Boundary Campground.

INTRODUCTION Tucked away in a lesser used corner of the Wallowa Mountains, this loop provides an excellent opportunity for experienced hikers to explore some outstanding country, see plenty of wildlife, and enjoy lonesome trails. Although there is only one lake along the way, anglers have ample opportunity to try their luck catching Bear Creek's many brook and rainbow trout. (Artificial flies or lures are required, and any bull trout must be released unharmed.) The hike also features two historic log cabins, both of which are worth exploring. This trip's main attraction, however, at least from a scenery standpoint, is the spectacular hike along Washboard Ridge, one of the most outstanding ridge walks in Oregon. Although the views are awe inspiring, the hike is quite rugged, so only fit hikers should consider this trip.

DESCRIPTION The well-used Bear Creek Trail goes south, paralleling the cascading waters of boulder-strewn Bear Creek through an open forest of western larches, Engelmann spruces, grand firs, ponderosa pines, and Douglas firs. A few stately black cottonwoods grow near the stream along with several shrubs, including wild rose, thimbleberry, snowberry, alder, birch, and vine maple. After 0.2 mile cross the creek on a bridge beneath moss-draped cliffs. The trail then closely follows the stream for almost 1 mile through dense riparian vegetation. The trail then climbs a bit to a cliff-edged bluff overlooking the stream before dropping to a pleasant creekside campsite at 1.8 miles.

At 2.1 miles you hop over the trickle of water in Baker Gulch, after which you gradually ascend in open forest with occasional views of the wooded ridges to the south and west. By 3.3 miles you drop back down to Bear Creek and pass two good campsites. Then it's another mile to a large meadow with a cluster of landmarks: first a junction with Goat Creek Trail (go straight), then a bridge over that trail's namesake creek, and finally a spacious and inviting camping area in the trees at the meadow's south end. Just 0.4 mile past this camp is an unsigned but obvious spur trail that goes right 150 yards to the beautifully built log structure of the old Bear Creek Guard Station. This historic cabin is now locked, but there are good camps nearby and use trails that lead to Bear Creek for water.

Back on Bear Creek Trail, it's another 0.4 mile before you come to a junction at the start of the loop. Turn right and, 120 yards later, encounter an easy ford of Bear Creek, which after mid-July probably won't even get your ankles wet.

To this point the hike has been very easy, but the gentle creekside ramble is now over, as you rapidly ascend the western side of Bear Creek Canyon. The mostly open slopes here are surprisingly dry, hosting both western juniper and mountain mahogany, species that are normally found in the desert mountains of southeastern Oregon, not in the relatively wet Wallowa Mountains. In addition to botanical interest, these slopes provide nice views of the Bear Creek drainage and the high peaks at the stream's headwaters.

The first mile of steady uphill includes six switchbacks to ease the steepness somewhat, but the ascent is still a challenge for both thighs and calves. At 1.4 miles from the Bear Creek ford you cross Dobbin Creek, whose cool, rapidly falling waters are a welcome relief from the heat of the climb. The next mile uses numerous short switchbacks to climb through a shady forest, where the trail is often overgrown with a mix of thimbleberry, gooseberry, currant, bracken fern, tall larkspur, coneflower, cow parsnip, bluebells, false Solomon's seal, and (beware) stinging nettle. The uphill is unrelenting, but the shade makes things more comfortable. That shady comfort comes to an abrupt halt at 2.4 miles from Bear Creek when you enter a sea of snags left by the old Fox Point Fire.

Warning: *Deadfall is sometimes a problem in this area.*

Regrowing trees were only a few feet tall as of 2006, so don't expect any shade. In the meantime though, taking advantage of the sun are several species of wildflowers. Look for abundant July blossoms of false hellebore, aster, Lewis' monkeyflower, penstemon, pearly everlasting, and paintbrush, among others. After a little less than 1 mile of uphill walking through the burn, you pass a marshy pond backed by a red-tinged ridge. You then climb a bit more before finally returning to unburned forest shortly before a junction.

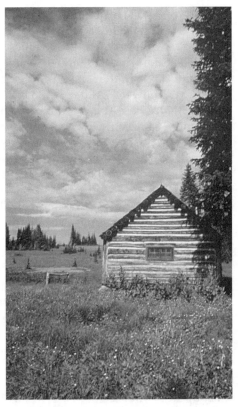

Standley Cabin

Turn left on a well-used trail and go gradually uphill for 1 mile through forest and rolling ridgetop meadows to Standley Cabin. This quaint log cabin, which formerly served as a Forest Service guard station, is now locked, but it is fun to poke around the outside and take pictures. There is a tiny but reliable spring nearby, which feeds a creek that flows through a lush green meadow. Camping is banned within 50 yards of the spring, but there are plenty of legal sites nearby.

About 0.1 mile south of Standley Cabin the trail forks. Bear left, following signs to Upper Bear Creek, and begin perhaps the most magnificent ridge walk in Oregon. Following Washboard Ridge for its entire length, the route starts high and remains so, never dipping below 7300 feet and topping out at over 8000. The views are tremendous, especially west across the great depths of the Minam River

Canyon to the distant Elkhorn Mountains, and southeast to the highest peaks of the Wallowa Mountains. Trees rarely block the view, with only a few scattered whitebark pines, subalpine firs, and mountain hemlocks. Gentle breezes (and occasionally strong winds) help to keep you comfortable in the hot sun and create waves in the acres of grasses and wildflowers. And there are plenty of wildflowers to blow around, with fine displays of lupine, Cusick's speedwell, buckwheat, penstemon, campion, yarrow, orange mountain dandelion, and other blossoms that usually peak in mid-July. All in all it is great fun. But that fun is reserved for hardy and experienced backpackers, because the trail is often very faint—frequently disappearing in the meadows—and Washboard Ridge is true to its name, with lots of ups and downs. The trail is also steep and narrow in places, making it dangerous for stock, although horses sometimes use it.

The first mile is all uphill on the west side of the ridge, as the trail ascends a huge meadow where the tread soon disappears. There are a few large cairns to guide you, but they are surprisingly hard to find. The best plan is to angle uphill to the southeast until you meet the tread again just below the ridgecrest. Now on clearer trail, descend a steep section with impressive views of the knife-edge ridge ahead and the Minam River Canyon below. Wildlife frequent this area. Two common species to look for are Rocky Mountain elk and calliope hummingbirds—the first is Oregon's largest wild mammal and the latter its smallest bird. You can also expect families of blue grouse to suddenly flush up from your feet, often in a startling flurry of activity.

The next 2 miles stay almost exclusively on the west side of the ridge, with easterly views only at the few places where you hit saddles. The most notable feature of this section, however, is that it can be rather scary for hikers who are afraid of heights. In several places the rocky and dangerously sloping trail cuts across dizzying ledges that are frequently no more than a foot across. So even though the views are distracting, keep a close eye on your footing. After negotiating this section, an easier (but no less scenic) segment follows as the trail goes through long grassy saddles and rolling ridgetop meadows.

At 4.8 miles from Standley Cabin you pass 50 feet above a tiny spring (the first potential water along the ridge) and, 30 yards later, come to a junction with the Miner Basin Trail. Go straight and then cut across the steep slopes of Bald Mountain before traversing a large sloping meadow, where, once again, the tread fades away. The proper route goes downhill and then traverses a long basin on the west side of Washboard Ridge. If you lose the tread, simply head toward Sturgill Saddle, an obvious low point in the ridge a little over 1 mile to the southeast. Once you are there, the tread becomes obvious again as it drops into an exceptionally scenic alpine basin beneath an unnamed 8352-foot peak. Alpine buttercups, Cusick's speedwell, pink heather, and other alpine wildflowers seem to be everywhere, and small creeks provide much-needed water. There are several places to camp here and you will probably have the basin all to yourself.

From the south end of this basin the trail climbs 500 feet to 8100-foot Sandy Saddle and then turns left (east) and follows a ridge. The route initially contours but soon begins descending, steeply at times, to a meadow-filled saddle. This place has no official name, but it is locally referred to as Bear Saddle. Although the trail disappears here, it is easy to make your way east across the meadow to an obvious cairn marking the junction with Bear Creek Trail.

Several trails converge at this remote location. To the right (south), hikers with extra time could spend several days exploring such worthwhile destinations as Wilson Basin and North Minam Meadows. Another option is to go straight (east) on an initially promising use path that heads uphill toward Bear Lake. Unfortunately, this trail soon disappears, forcing hikers to make a rather rugged scramble to that lake. Two trails go to the left at Bear Saddle, neither of which is initially easy to see. The one angling slightly left is the official trail to Bear Lake. The tread of this path becomes obvious about 100 feet from the junction as

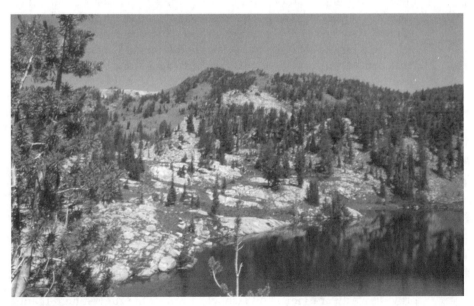

Bear Lake

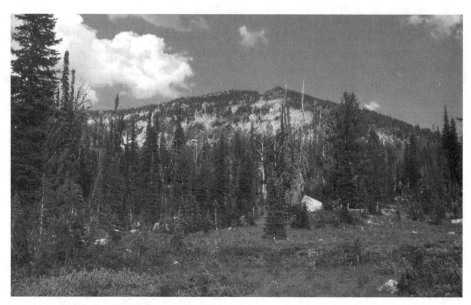

Above the headwaters of Bear Creek

it contours and then climbs sharply for 0.6 mile to the shores of clear, 20-foot-deep Bear Lake. This lovely 10-acre pool is ideal for fishing (it's filled with hungry brook trout), swimming (if you don't mind chilly water), and camping (with a good site above the north side of the outlet creek).

The return route of the recommended loop goes sharply left at the Bear Saddle junction. The tread is initially hidden in meadow but becomes obvious after about 50 yards. After 0.2 mile the trail crosses the outlet of Bear Lake and then descends 15 well-graded switchbacks through an area covered with white-granite boulders to the bottom of Bear Creek Canyon. For the next 1.5 miles the trail stays on the forested hillside above the stream, although from time to time you can see meadows below you beside the creek.

Tip: *Look for herds of elk in these meadows, especially early in the morning.*

After this traverse, four lazy switchbacks take you down to the creek and, at 4.5 miles from Bear Saddle, to Middle Bear Camp, a nice spot in the trees at the south end of a small but particularly inviting meadow.

Below Middle Bear Camp the hiking is easy and enjoyable, although views are infrequent through the forest. Occasional meadows provide westward views to Washboard Ridge, the rugged high points of which you will recognize from earlier in the trip. A little over 2 miles below Middle Bear Camp is a rock-hop crossing of Granite Creek, after which you continue mostly downhill, often in large sloping meadows. Deer frequently browse in these meadows and ground squirrels squeak loud alarms at your passing. In the forested sections between the meadows, look for snowshoe hares bounding away with their summer-brown bodies and flashing white back feet.

At 8.5 miles from Bear Saddle you pass two small cairns on your left that mark the junction with Miner Basin Trail. Go straight on the main trail and, a little less than 1 mile later, pass two unsigned trails that drop to pleasant campsites near Bear Creek. At 13.4 miles from Bear Saddle, although the distance seems less than that with all the easy downhill, you return to the junction with the trail to Standley Cabin and the close of your loop. Go straight and retrace your steps back to your car.

POSSIBLE ITINERARY			
	Camp	Miles	Elevation Gain
Day 1	Standley Cabin	9.6	3700
Day 2	Basin below Sturgill Saddle	8.0	1800
Day 3	Middle Bear Camp (with		
	side trip to Bear Lake)	8.0	1000
Day 4	Out	14.0	300

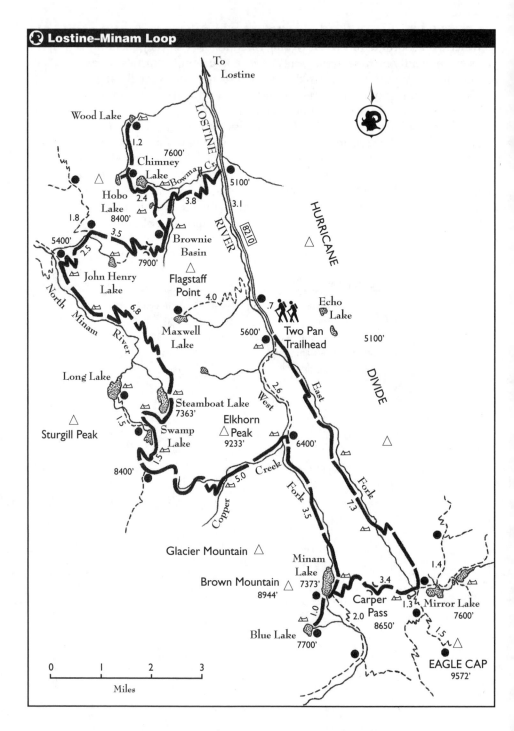

To
Lostine

Wood Lake

1.2

7600'

Chimney
Lake

LOSTINE

Bowman Cr.

5100'

2.4

3.8

3.1

8210

HURRICANE

Hobo
Lake

8400'

1.8

3.5

5400'

2.5

Brownie
Basin

7900'

RIVER

John Henry
Lake

6.8

Flagstaff
Point

4.0

Maxwell
Lake

.7

Echo
Lake

Two Pan
Trailhead

5600'

5100'

North Minam River

DIVIDE

Long Lake

Steamboat Lake
7363'

West

East

2.6

Sturgill Peak

1.5

Swamp
Lake

Elkhorn
Peak
9233'

6400'

Fork

Fork

7.3

8400'

1.5

Copper

5.0

Creek

Fork

3.5

Glacier Mountain

1.4

Brown Mountain
8944'

Minam
Lake
7373'

3.4

1.3

1.0

2.0

Carper
Pass
8650'

Mirror Lake
7600'

Blue Lake
7700'

1.5

EAGLE CAP
9572'

0   1   2   3
Miles

20 Lostine–Minam Loop

RATINGS (1–10)			MILES	ELEVATION GAIN	DAYS	SHUTTLE MILEAGE
Scenery	Solitude	Difficulty	43	8700	4–6	N/A
9	4	6	(52)	(11,000)	(5–8)	

MAP   Imus Geographics—*Wallowa Mountains*

USUALLY OPEN   July to October

BEST   Late July to September

PERMITS   Yes (free and unlimited)

RULES   No fires within 0.25 mile of Chimney, Laverty, Mirror, Moccasin, Steamboat, or Swamp lakes; maximum group size of 6 people/9 stock in Lakes Basin and at Minam and Blue lakes

CONTACT   Wallowa Valley visitor center, (541) 426-4978

SPECIAL ATTRACTIONS   Great mountain scenery

PROBLEMS   Crowded in spots; short road walk; unbridged stream crossings; thunderstorms

HOW TO GET THERE   Drive Highway 82 east from La Grande to the community of Lostine. Turn south on a paved road signed LOSTINE RIVER CAMPGROUNDS. The road turns to gravel after 7 miles and becomes Forest Road 8210. The route gets rougher and more bumpy as it goes up the canyon, but remains passable for passenger cars. Reach the Bowman Trailhead some 15 miles from Lostine. If you have two cars, leave one here and the other 3.8 miles further south at the spacious Two Pan Trailhead.

INTRODUCTION   This is one of several classic loop hikes in the Wallowa Mountains. Like the others, this one includes all the major attractions of this wonderful range. There are mountain lakes, alpine passes, wildflower-filled meadows, clear streams, and granite peaks. These features make this hike fairly popular, but it's not as crowded as the Wallowa River Loop (Trip 21). For those with less time or ambition, this route lends itself nicely to a shorter version. In fact, the most common way this trip is done skips East Lostine Canyon and Minam Lake and heads directly up the West Lostine River to the Copper Creek Trail. Without side trips this alternate loop is only about 32 miles long. Don't forget your fishing gear (lots of lake and stream fishing is available), binoculars (to search for elk, bighorn sheep, and mountain goats), swim suit, and, most of all, your camera (the scenery is terrific).

DESCRIPTION   From Two Pan Trailhead hike up the trail for 0.1 mile to a junction. The short version of this loop goes to the right. For a longer, more satisfying trip, keep left on the popular East Fork Lostine River Trail. The wide path makes a moderately steep climb through forests for the first 2.5 miles as it ascends toward the stream's high glacial valley. Views become more impressive near the top of the climb, especially of imposing Hurricane Divide to the east. All that climbing is rewarded when you enter the impressive glacier-carved upper East Lostine River Valley. Jagged ridges rise steeply on either side, while the crystalline river flows lazily through wildflower meadows on the valley floor. At the 3.2-mile point a large, swampy, wide spot in the stream goes by the name of Lost "Lake."

For the next few miles the trail remains nearly level as it wanders up this beautiful valley.

> *Tip:* Look for elk, deer, and mountain goats in this area, especially in the early morning and evening.

You are walking through a classic U-shaped glacial canyon, which adds geologic interest to the fine scenery. The trail travels through a delightful mix of open forests, meadows, and boulder fields. At the head of the valley looms the distinctive shape of Eagle Cap.

Cross the stream near the head of the valley and increase the rate of your climb as you switchback through open forests to a four-way junction. Most visitors turn left here to visit lovely Mirror Lake—well worth a side trip. Your route, however, turns right, passing below Upper Lake and providing excellent views down the East Lostine Canyon. If you choose to camp in this popular but fragile basin, be even more careful that usual to leave no trace. The trail now begins a moderately steep climb toward Carper Pass. Frequent views of Eagle Cap, resembling Yosemite's Half Dome from this angle, make the climb more of a joy than a strain. As expected, the views from the pass are exceptional. From the high point the trail makes a rolling descent before dropping more consistently to the south end of large Minam Lake.

An earthen dam blocks this lake's former outlet to the south, so it now drains principally north into the West Lostine River. Aptly named Brown Mountain dominates the skyline to the west.

To continue your tour, turn north as the trail loops around the east shore of Minam Lake and then gradually descends the valley of the West Lostine River. If the scenery in the East Lostine Valley rates a 10, then the West Lostine has to be a 9.9. You cross the stream twice as you wind down through the meadows and forests of this lovely valley. There are no bridges, so be prepared to wade (chilly, but not dangerous).

About 3.5 miles from Minam Lake is a poorly marked junction at a talus slope. Turn left on the Copper Creek Trail to a ford of the West Lostine River. There are good camps in the meadows nearby. The trail then begins to climb up the valley of Copper Creek crossing the stream four times along the way.

Although the climb is moderate in grade, it seems to go on forever. However, the excellent scenery is ample compensation. Camps are abundant in this section of bouldery areas and meadows, with a terrific variety of wildflowers throughout the summer.

Eventually the trail veers away from the creek and climbs to a high, sandy plateau. In the basin to the right is Swamp Lake. More distant

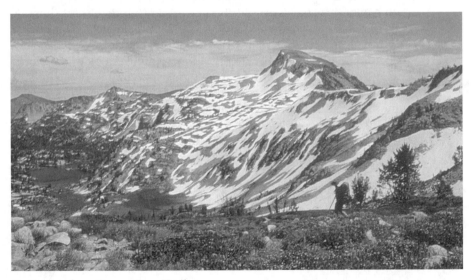

Eagle Cap from Carper Pass Trail

views extend to the Matterhorn, Eagle Cap, and the other distinctive peaks of this range. Now the trail gradually loses a bit of elevation to a junction where you turn right. This route makes a long, switchbacking descent into the meadowy basin holding Swamp Lake, which has good camps near the north end. The south end of this irregularly shaped pool is an intricate mix of meadows, creeks, and small ponds that looks like a Japanese garden.

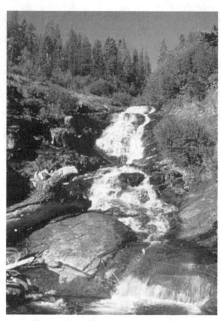

Falls along Bowman Creek

Tip: A side trail drops from here to large Long Lake, which features secluded camps and good fishing, but has only limited views.

To continue your tour, top a low saddle near two small ponds (good camps) and enjoy a nice view down to Steamboat Lake. The route makes a series of switchbacks down a mostly open slope to the south end of this lake, where the best camps are along the east shore. A large rock island apparently looked like a steamboat to imaginative early travelers. The trail veers away from Steamboat Lake over a low rise before descending through a meadow to an overlook of the North Minam River Canyon. For the next few miles the trail leads down into this canyon in a series of irregular switchbacks over semi-open terrain. Numerous side creeks provide ample water. Several good campsites highlight the last couple of miles of the descent as the trail follows an attractive stream to spacious North Minam Meadows.

Tip: Although the trail skirts this large meadow, it is worthwhile to walk over for a visit.

Near the north end of the meadow you turn right at a junction with the Bowman Trail. Climb in a series of moderately steep switchbacks, enjoying several nice views down to North Minam Meadows along the way. You pass an unseen waterfall and then reach a junction with the Bear Creek Trail. Keep right and 1.2 miles later look for the unsigned and unmaintained path to John Henry Lake. The lake, 0.5 mile away, features nice camps.

The main trail climbs to Wilson Pass, where there is an excellent view to the east of Twin Peaks and the Hurricane Divide. Your route then switchbacks down to the trees above Brownie Basin, a long, scenic meadow with a lovely setting which is well worth a visit. The trail goes north along the slope above the meadow to a junction. Here you have the option of either heading directly out to your car, or investing a bit more time and energy in the worthwhile side trip to Chimney and Hobo lakes.

To do the side trip, keep left at the junction, traverse a view-packed slope to Laverty Lake, and then round a ridge to large and beautiful Chimney Lake. Granite peaks rise to the west and two small islands add to the scene. To reach the more alpine setting of Hobo Lake, climb above Chimney Lake to a saddle. From here turn left at a junction and climb over rocky meadows to the high basin holding Hobo Lake.

Tip: Ambitious hikers can also make the the cross-country scramble to the views from atop Lookout Mountain and take the trail down to the lovely meadow basin holding Wood Lake.

Back at Brownie Basin, the well-graded trail crosses Bowman Creek and then drops in long gentle switchbacks to the Lostine River Road. Near the bottom, a nice sloping waterfall on the creek adds scenic interest. From the Bowman Trailhead it's an easy 3.8-mile walk up the road to Two Pan Trailhead and your car. (So easy, in fact, you may be able to talk your companion into doing the extra walk, while you volunteer for the "difficult" task of guarding the packs and daydreaming about this wonderful trip.)

POSSIBLE ITINERARY			
	Camp	Miles	Elevation Gain
Day 1	Mirror Lake	7.3	2100
Day 2	Minam Lake (with side trip to Blue Lake)	5.4	1500
Day 3	Swamp Lake	10.0	2200
Day 4	John Henry Lake	11.1	2000
Day 5	Brownie Basin (with side trip to Chimney, Hobo, and Wood lakes)	9.7	2600
Day 6	Out (with road walk to Two Pan Trailhead)	7.6	600

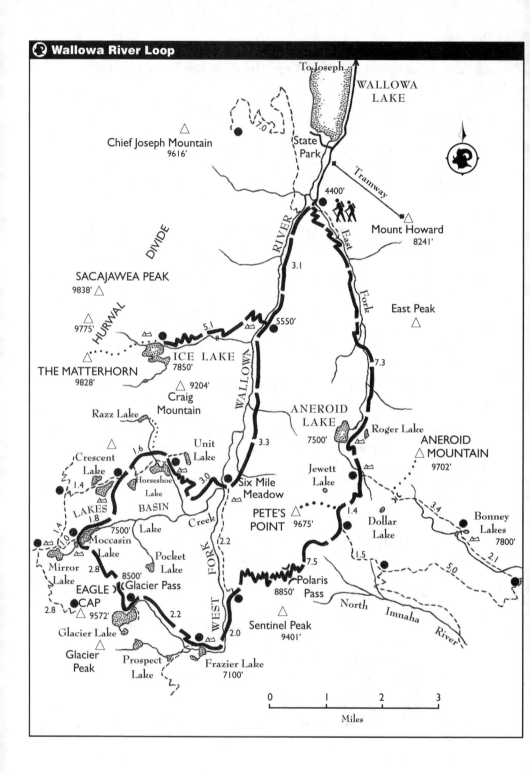

21 Wallowa River Loop

RATINGS (1–10)			MILES	ELEVATION GAIN	DAYS	SHUTTLE MILEAGE
Scenery	Solitude	Difficulty				
10	2	7	36	7100	4–5	N/A
			(54)	(11,700)	(5–10)	

MAP Imus Geographics—*Wallowa Mountains*

USUALLY OPEN July to October

BEST Late July and August

PERMITS Yes (free and unlimited)

RULES No fires within 0.25 mile of Glacier, Mirror, Moccasin, or Upper lakes; maximum group size of 6 people/9 stock in Lakes Basin and at Ice Lake

CONTACT Wallowa Valley visitor center, (541) 426-4978

SPECIAL ATTRACTIONS Stunning mountain scenery

PROBLEMS Crowded; thunderstorms; horse-pounded trails

HOW TO GET THERE Drive east on Highway 82 from La Grande for 70 miles to Joseph. Continue south to Wallowa Lake and the huge trail-head parking lot at the south end of this scenic lake.

INTRODUCTION This trip features the best scenery in the most beautiful mountains in Oregon. Crystal-clear lakes and streams, meadows filled with wildflowers, glacier-polished white granite peaks . . . the list of joys excites the imagination, and the reality lives up to those high expectations. Unfortunately, the trails here are also the most popular in the Eagle Cap Wilderness, traveled by thousands of hikers and horses. However, the beauty more than compensates for the aggravation.

DESCRIPTION Go left on the East Fork Wallowa River Trail, following signs to Aneroid Lake. You switchback up the mostly forested hillside and after 1.6 miles pass a small waterfall and a water diversion dam. The trail enters the official wilderness just beyond this point. Continue climbing at a gentler pace and enter the stream's more level upper valley. As the trail leads upstream, views of meadows and the surrounding peaks become more frequent and enticing. Cross the stream on a footbridge 3.9 miles from the trailhead and continue up its east bank, eventually reaching the shores of large and very scenic Aneroid Lake. Good though sometimes crowded camps abound in the woods nearby.

This lake makes an excellent base camp for exploring the highly scenic terrain nearby. Don't miss the easy stroll around the lake itself—including a stop at the privately owned cabins at the lake's south end. A much more strenuous option is the scramble to the top of Aneroid Mountain (a long, tiring, trailless climb, but *what a view!*). Another worthwhile trip is Dollar Lake and the easy climb up the ridge behind it. Jewett Lake, on a bench southwest of Aneroid Lake, is also worth a visit. Highly recommended are the lovely Bonney Lakes and a magnificent 15-mile wildflower loop around a ridge south of these lakes. Finally, the climb to the summit of Pete's Point is extremely rewarding. This peak is most easily reached by a sketchy boot path that climbs steeply up the exposed ridge on the peak's northeast side.

Once you've sampled the dayhike possibilities from Aneroid Lake, pack up your gear and continue south. The trail climbs through a typically glorious Wallowa Mountains meadow on the way to exposed Tenderfoot Pass. The trail then traverses a slope and climbs to the fine view from Polaris Pass.

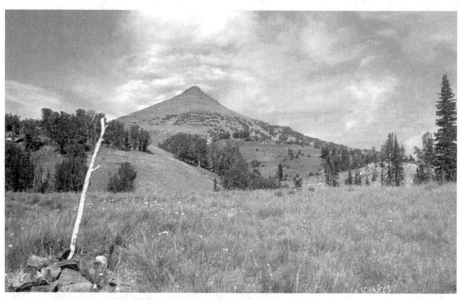

Aneroid Mountain from the southwest

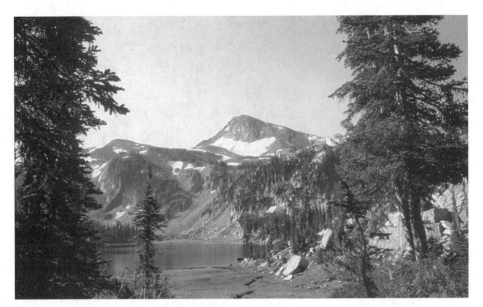

Mirror Lake and Eagle Cap

Warning: *The trail to Polaris Pass receives only irregular maintenance.*

The view west from this grandstand is stunning, as most of the rugged Wallowa Mountains spread out in front of you. From the pass the trail drops almost 2000 feet in a seemingly endless series of very gradual switchbacks all the way to the bottom of the valley. There is no water on the long descent, which explains why this loop is less attractive in the opposite direction.

Once you reach the bottom, turn left (upstream) at the junction with the West Fork Wallowa River Trail and soon enter the highly scenic upper valley of this stream. Cross the creek—there is no bridge, so expect a chilly wade—and continue another mile to the good camps at scenic Frazier Lake.

Tip: *A nice side trip from Frazier Lake leads south past beautiful Little Frazier Lake to the view from Hawkins Pass—2.3 miles from Frazier Lake.*

The trail now climbs a series of meadowy benches beside the waterfalls and cascades of the West Fork Wallowa River to Glacier Lake—one of the classic beauty spots in the state of Oregon. Camping here is *not* recommended due to the fragile alpine terrain and the exposed nature of camps.

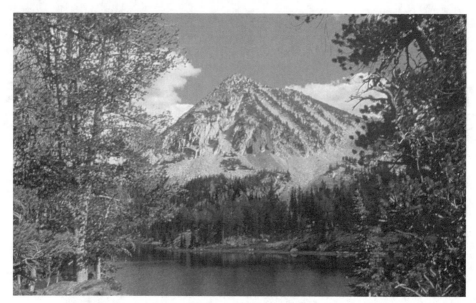

Craig Mountain over Ice Lake

Warning: *The water of this aptly named lake is bone-chillingly cold even on the hottest days of summer.*

Tip: *While views across any part of Glacier Lake are terrific, perhaps the best is from the east shore looking toward Eagle Cap and Glacier Peak. Reach this view by crossing the outlet creek and following a use path beside the lake for a few hundred yards.*

Once you manage to pull yourself away from the beauty of Glacier Lake, climb in a series of short switchbacks to the tremendous view from windswept Glacier Pass. Spread out to the north are the forested Lakes Basin and myriad distant peaks. Spend some time here to rest and pick out the many landmarks.

The trail now drops 1200 feet into the Lakes Basin, a heavily used area that consists of a series of large, beautiful lakes that seem to pop up at every turn in the trail. Every lake features a different view of the surrounding peaks. The first one you'll reach is Moccasin Lake, perhaps the most scenic of all, where there are numerous excellent camps (as is true at all of the lakes). Side trips abound but the easy stroll to Mirror Lake and tiny Upper Lake should be included in any itinerary. More ambitious hikers can follow exposed but view-packed routes to Carper Pass or even the top of Eagle Cap.

Tip: A superior but unmarked and hard-to-find side trail leads from the east end of Moccasin Lake to the austere setting of Pocket Lake.

To continue the loop trip, turn right at Moccasin Lake and take Trail #1810A. Pass Douglas Lake, with an unnamed but spectacular granite ridge for a backdrop, and then Lee and Horseshoe lakes as you slowly descend through the Lakes Basin. Side trips from Horseshoe Lake lead to forest-rimmed Unit Lake or lovely Razz Lake (the trail to the latter is not marked or maintained). Reluctantly, you must now leave the Lakes Basin and descend through forest to the West Fork Wallowa River. Several moderate switchbacks eventually lead down to a stream crossing just before you enter Six Mile Meadow (good camps). Turn left at the trail junction here and follow the river downstream as you gradually leave the high country behind. There are several nice cross-canyon views, and small side creeks provide water.

If time and energy allow, a highly recommended side trip switchbacks up to Ice Lake—located in a high basin on the Hurwal Divide to the west. This large, scenic lake provides a good base camp for scrambles up The Matterhorn and Sacajawea Peak, the highest summits in the Wallowa Mountains. Other rewarding pursuits there include angling, scanning for the area's mountain goats, and simply sitting and enjoying the scenery. To reach Ice Lake, leave the main trail 3.3 miles north of Six Mile Meadow and turn left on a path that climbs a seemingly endless series of switchbacks to the lake. The tedium of this climb is broken by ever-improving views and a terrific look at a long waterfall on Adams Creek.

Once you convince yourself to leave this paradise, return down all those switchbacks to the West Fork Wallowa River Trail. Turn north and follow this woodsy path back down to your car.

POSSIBLE ITINERARY			
	Camp	Miles	Elevation Gain
Day 1	Aneroid Lake	6.3	3200
Day 2	Aneroid Lake (dayhike up Pete's Point)	8.0	2300
Day 3	Frazier Lake	11.8	2200
Day 4	Horseshoe Lake	8.5	1500
Day 5	Ice Lake	11.1	2400
Day 6	Out	8.2	100

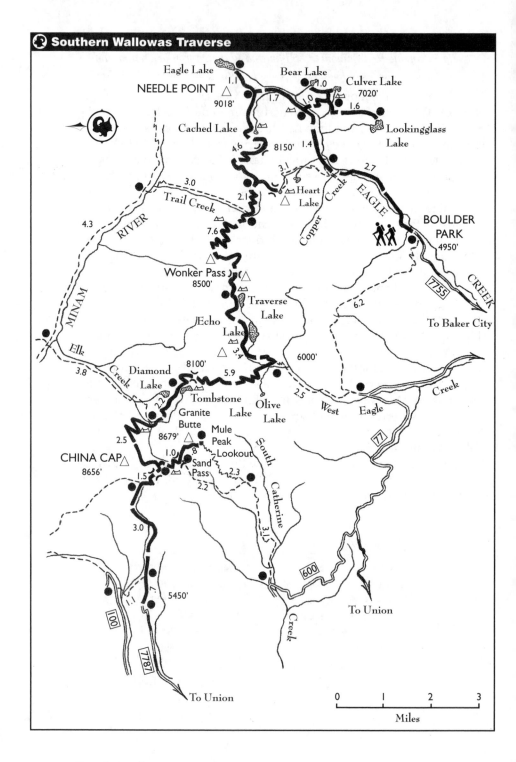

Eagle Lake

Bear Lake

NEEDLE POINT
1.1
9018'

1.0

Culver Lake
7020'

1.7

1.0

1.6

Cached Lake

4.6

8150'

1.4

Lookingglass
Lake

3.1

2.7

Trail Creek

3.0

Heart
Lake

Copper Creek

EAGLE

2.1

RIVER

BOULDER
PARK
4950'

4.3

7.6

Wonker Pass
8500'

MINAM

Traverse
Lake

Elk

Echo
Lake

6.2

7755

CREEK

To Baker City

Diamond
Lake

3.8

8100'

3.4

Creek

2.2

Tombstone

5.9

6000'

2.5

West Eagle

Creek

Olive
Lake

Granite
Butte

Lake

77

2.5

8679'

Mule
Peak
Lookout

CHINA CAP
8656'

1.0

8

South Catherine

1.5

Sand
Pass

2.3

2.2

3.1

3.0

600

00

.7

5450'

1.1

7787

Creek

To Union

To Union

0   1   2   3

Miles

22 Southern Wallowas Traverse

RATINGS (1–10)			MILES	ELEVATION GAIN	DAYS	SHUTTLE MILEAGE
Scenery	Solitude	Difficulty				
9	6	8	40	9400	4–5	42
			(55)	(13,400)	(6–8)	

MAP Imus Geographics—*Wallowa Mountains*

USUALLY OPEN July to October

BEST Mid-July to early August

PERMITS Yes (free and unlimited)

RULES No fires within 0.25 mile of Eagle Lake; maximum group size of 12 people/18 stock

CONTACT Wallowa Valley visitor center, (541) 426-4978

SPECIAL ATTRACTIONS Mountain scenery; relative solitude

PROBLEMS Rugged up-and-down hike; thunderstorms

HOW TO GET THERE The east trailhead is at Boulder Park, a former horse-outfitting ranch on Eagle Creek. Begin from Highway 203 just south of the village of Medical Springs. Turn east at a fork, following signs for Tamarack Campground. After 1.7 miles turn left on Forest Road 67. In 13 miles, just before a bridge over Eagle Creek, turn left on Road 77. After another 0.7 mile keep right at a fork and travel on Road 7755 for 3.5 miles to the roadend trailhead. The west trailhead is reached by turning east on Forest Road 7785 off Highway 203 about 8 miles north of Medical Springs. This gravel road follows the North Fork of Catherine Creek for 3.5 miles to a fork. Turn right on Road 7787 to the Buck Creek Trailhead.

INTRODUCTION The southern Wallowa Mountains are both very similar to and quite different from the northern part of the range. As in the areas to the north, the scenery is spectacular, with the same enchanting combination of granite peaks, alpine lakes, and wildflowers. The southern part, however, has a very different character. First of all, the trail population is smaller. While you won't be lonesome, longer road access

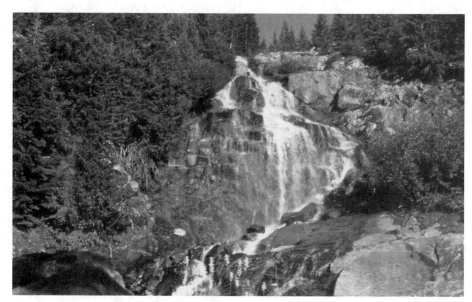

Copper Creek Falls

and more rugged trails mean far fewer people choose to hike in this region. The terrain also differs from the northern Wallowas. Granite peaks are still found in abundance, but the geology here is more varied, with many prominent peaks being more reddish than white. Finally, the forests are more open and the meadows more expansive, so vistas are wider and more common. This attractive but difficult hike traces a rugged up-and-down route as it alternates between the high passes and deep canyons that characterize the southern Wallowas. For the fit hiker who longs for the beauty of the Wallowas without the crowds, this is a wonderful choice. The hike is described here from east to west.

DESCRIPTION   Begin by hiking northeast up an abandoned jeep road across the remains of a landslide to a bridged crossing of Eagle Creek. Now a pleasant footpath, the route climbs through forests as it closely parallels the stream. You recross Eagle Creek and soon reach the ford of Copper Creek—expect to get your feet wet until late summer—just downstream from impressive Copper Creek Falls.

> *Tip:* For the best view of this falls take a short spur trail north of the creek.

Keep straight at a trail junction a little past Copper Creek, sticking with the Eagle Creek Trail. The trail gets rougher but the terrain is more open, with meadows and views of the surrounding peaks. At 4.1 miles is large Eagle Meadows, with good camps. There is also a junction here with the route to Lookingglass Lake.

To visit the lovely lakes in the high cirques to the south and east, ford Eagle Creek and climb a fairly steep trail up the canyon wall. Views to the north of Needle Point and the basin of Eagle Lake improve as you ascend to a trail junction near the base of a meadow. To the right, a 1.6-mile trail climbs over a mostly open ridge before dropping a bit to large Lookingglass Lake. This deep lake has good fishing but is artificially dammed, so when the water is lower it resembles a bathtub. The rocky terrain around the lake makes for generally poor camping but the views are excellent. Back at the last junction, the left fork quickly enters the basin holding very scenic Culver Lake. Towering cliffs behind the east shore of this lake present a challenge for even the widest-angle camera lens. The trail continues north another mile to Bear Lake. This pool is attractive, but less spectacular than Culver or Lookingglass lakes.

Tip: *The best plan is to camp down at Eagle Meadows and dayhike up to these lakes.*

Continuing north on the Eagle Creek Trail, wildflowers brighten the canyon ascent as the scenery changes from meadows and open slopes back into forest. Not long after the trail begins to make a switchbacking climb is a rock cairn (and possibly a sign) marking the junction with the trail to Eagle Lake. Although Eagle Lake is artificially dammed and has generally poor campsites, it's still well worth the side trip. The last 0.3 mile of the trail to this lake is up a steep granite ridge with stunted whitebark pines framing excellent views back down the canyon. The lake itself sits in a spectacular alpine basin rimmed by 9,000-foot granite peaks. There are few trees in this high bowl, but the scenery is impressive.

For better camps, return to the main trail and climb to the meadow flat holding tiny Cached Lake. Nice sheltered camps are in the trees on this pool's north side.

Tip: *Be sure to walk around to the lake's southwest shore for some excellent views across Cached Lake to Needle Point—dominating the local skyline.*

As is true in many parts of the Wallowas, friendly deer are likely to visit your camp in the evening.

Tip: *"Peak baggers" will want to make the steep, but not technically difficult, scramble to the top of Needle Point. The view from the summit is truly outstanding, especially of the deep, curving Minam River Canyon to the north.*

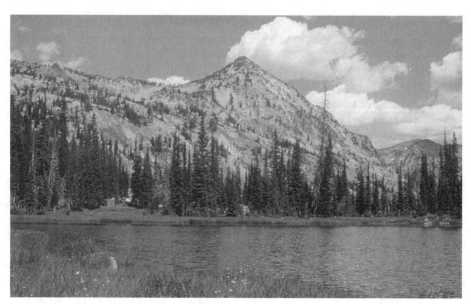
Needle Point over Cached Lake

From Cached Lake your trail makes a long looping climb to a windswept pass and then descends back into forest to a meadow with a trail junction. An excellent side trip turns left here, climbs steeply over a rocky pass, and drops to the alpine cirque holding tiny Arrow Lake. With a high granite peak, small islands, and a rocky wildflower meadow, Arrow Lake is a magical place. Now you return to the main trail and switchback steadily downhill to Trail Creek. You'll have to get used to this pattern of alternating between high passes and deep canyons because that pretty much describes the rest of this trip. There are precious few stretches of level trail. Fortunately, frequent lakes and views provide ample compensation. A break in the trees partway down this particular descent provides an excellent view of the peaks to the west.

At the bottom of the canyon you go left at a junction and then cross Trail Creek. Rest for awhile and refill your water bottle before tackling the long 2300-foot climb to Wonker Pass. The well-graded trail climbs gradually for 1 mile to a nice meadow with a good campsite. From here you ascend through forest and then up a series of airy switchbacks on an exposed talus slope with increasingly good views to the pass.

From Wonker Pass it's only a short descent to the alpine basin holding beautiful Traverse Lake, with excellent camps. The lake has an idyllic setting in a large meadow surrounded by scattered islands of trees. The most impressive view is from the northwest shore looking back toward a prominent granite monolith beside Wonker Pass—*outstanding!*

To continue your tour, head away from the waters of Traverse Lake and soon reach a grand overlook of Echo Lake and the canyon below. (Yes, you're going *all the way down there.*) Walk past a nice spring and then drop to Echo Lake, which can be reached by any of several short side trails. A serrated ridge south of this lake makes a nice backdrop.

Warning: *Later in the summer, the water level drops in this artificially controlled lake making it much less attractive.*

You continue downhill, making a few switchbacks, and then cross a marshy area near a small pond. Switchbacks resume as the trail crosses semi-open slopes with high peaks on either side.

In a brushy area, long before the switchbacks end, is a junction. Turn right, cross the West Fork Eagle Creek, and brace yourself for the next big climb, as the trail regains all the previously lost elevation on a long and rather uneventful climb toward the pass above Tombstone Lake. There are nice views as you climb, but only intermittent shade. It's all worthwhile once you top out at a high pass because the views, as usual, are superb. From the pass the trail contours along a ridge for a bit then drops to the shores of Tombstone Lake, which has several choice camps for the weary hiker. The lake's name comes from a large

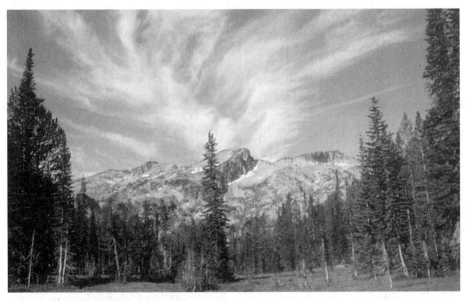

View west from Trail Creek Trail below Arrow Lake

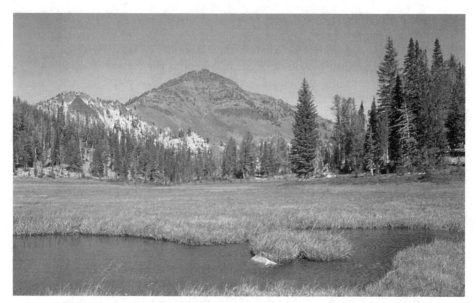

China Cap over meadow below Sand Pass

pinnacle rising from the southwestern shore. With some imagination, it might be said to resemble a tombstone.

The trail continues to the northwest, traveling above the basin holding woodsy Diamond Lake, which can be reached by steep side trails, and then continues to lose elevation to a trail junction beside Elk Creek. Turn left and cross the stream to an excellent campsite where two creeks meet. The meadow here is a lovely foreground for craggy Granite Butte to the south, and trees provide welcome shade.

Warning: *Bugs can be an annoyance here since the meadow is rather boggy.*

Leaving this meadow basin, you'll notice an older trail that climbs steeply up a slope to the left, but the well-graded newer trail climbs gradually to the right in two very long switchbacks with several good views along the way. Near the top of this climb the trail contours around sloping Burger Meadows and then climbs another hillside to a junction in the trees. For a quick exit, turn right, but keep straight for a terrific side trip.

The side trip first visits a beautiful meadow with a fine campsite, wildflowers, and small ponds. The view across this meadow toward prominent China Cap is particularly fetching. Leaving this meadow, you travel up very steep, sandy switchbacks to aptly named Sand Pass, often snowbound until late summer. Turn left at Sand Pass and follow a more gently graded trail that climbs through semi-open forest on a ridge east of Sand Pass. The way traverses an open slope a few hundred feet below the summit of Granite Butte and then crosses a saddle and goes up the spine of a narrow ridge to Mule Peak Lookout. This is one of Oregon's least visited fire lookouts, but the lack of visitors is due only to its isolation, because outstanding views extend in all directions. Fire-scarred forests below the peak testify to the need for this facility. The staff person here obviously has a good sense of humor, as signs identify this as the MULE PEAK BED & BREAFAST . . . PARKING IN THE REAR.

Back at the junction above Burger Meadows, turn west and climb to Burger Pass. The peaks on either side are not the typical white granite of the Wallowas but are reddish summits instead.

Tip: For those with energy to burn, the scramble up China Cap to the north is particularly rewarding.

The trail drops a few hundred feet to a junction below the pass. To the right is a long, view-packed ridge walk, but keep left to reach your car.

The final part of the hike is a pleasant downhill stretch, mostly in forest, along Middle Fork Catherine Creek. Keep straight at a trail junction near the bottom and soon reach the Buck Creek Trailhead—the close of an exhausting but glorious hike.

POSSIBLE ITINERARY

	Camp	Miles	Elevation Gain
Day 1	Eagle Meadows (with side trip to Lookingglass and Bear lakes)	11.3	2700
Day 2	Arrow Lake (with side trip to Eagle Lake)	9.6	3000
Day 3	Traverse Lake	10.8	2400
Day 4	Tombstone Lake	9.3	2200
Day 5	Meadow below Sand Pass (with side trip to Mule Peak Lookout)	7.8	2500
Day 6	Out	5.7	600

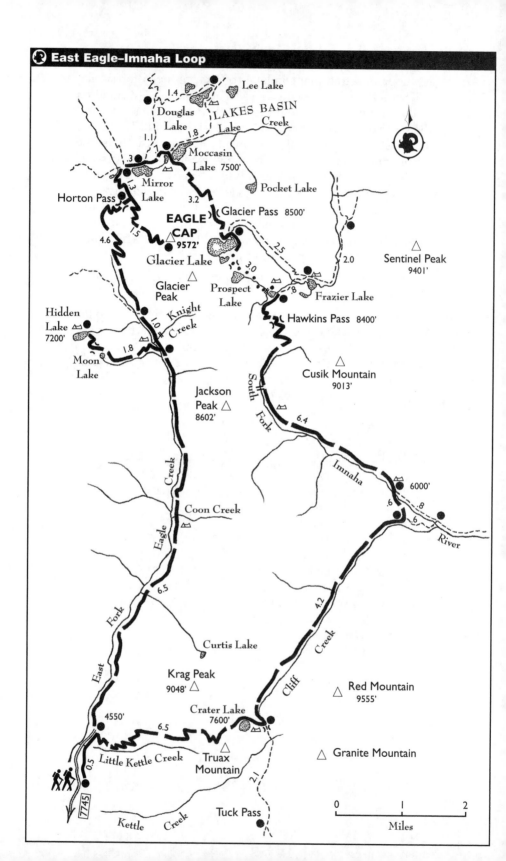

23 East Eagle–Imnaha Loop

RATINGS (1–10)			MILES	ELEVATION GAIN	DAYS	SHUTTLE MILEAGE
Scenery	Solitude	Difficulty	39	7900	5–6	N/A
10	4	6	(46)	(10,400)	(5–7)	

MAP Imus Geographics—*Wallowa Mountains*

USUALLY OPEN Mid-July to October

BEST Mid-July to August

PERMITS Yes (free and unlimited)

RULES No fires within 0.25 mile of Glacier, Mirror, Moccasin, or Sunshine lakes; maximum group size of 6 people/9 stock in Lakes Basin and at Frazier and Glacier lakes

CONTACT Wallowa Valley visitor center, (541) 426-4978

SPECIAL ATTRACTIONS Great mountain scenery; wildlife

PROBLEMS Crowded in spots; thunderstorms

HOW TO GET THERE To reach the start of this adventure, begin from Highway 203 just south of the village of Medical Springs. Turn east at a fork, following signs for Tamarack Campground. After 1.7 miles turn left on Forest Road 67. Drive for 13 miles, cross a bridge over Eagle Creek and then turn right on Road 77 past Tamarack Campground. After 6 miles turn left on Road 7745, following signs to the East Eagle Trailhead. Drive this gravel route for 5.3 miles to a recently constructed trailhead parking area on the right.

INTRODUCTION Here is yet another remarkably beautiful loop hike through the spectacular Wallowa Mountains. The focus here is on the southeast part of the range. As is true everywhere in these mountains, this trip features a wealth of breathtaking mountain scenery. The author's vocabulary of adjectives is simply inadequate to convey the glories. In the "Newspeak" language of George Orwell's *1984*, the scenery is "doubleplusgood."

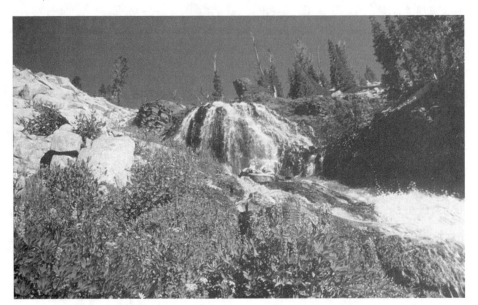

Falls below Prospect Lake

DESCRIPTION   From the new trailhead the path wanders through an attractive forest of beautiful old-growth ponderosa pine, grand fir, and western larch. You cross Little Kettle Creek and 0.5 mile from the trailhead, reach a junction with the Little Kettle Trail, the return leg of your loop. You go staight as the trail drops to creek level near the old trailhead. From here the route makes a gradual up-and-down climb with frequent views extending up 4000-foot canyon walls. Your way alternates among forests, brushy slopes, and meadows. Look for views of Krag Peak and several waterfalls across the canyon. Water from tributary creeks is abundant. There are limited camping opportunities in the lower canyon, although comfortable camps are possible a little south of Coon Creek and near Eagle Creek a bit farther along.

At 7.0 miles, a little before the waterfall on Knight Creek, is a possibly unsigned junction with the trail to Hidden Lake. To make this excellent side trip turn left and drop to a fairly easy ford of East Eagle Creek. There is a good campsite a bit further up the far bank. The trail climbs fairly steeply for about 1 mile before leveling off below Moon Lake. You climb over a low ridge and then drop down the other side to large and beautiful Hidden Lake. There are numerous excellent camps here as well as views of the craggy granite peaks circling the meadowy basin.

Tip: Some of the best views are from the lake's trailless north shore.

The lake also offers good fishing and swimming.

After returning to the East Eagle Trail, turn upstream and continue climbing. Keep right at the Frazier Pass junction as the trail gets narrower and rockier. Several long switchbacks moderate the climb. Cross East Eagle Creek and enter the high meadows of the headwall basin. Watch for deer and elk in this area. A long climb is required to exit this lovely basin as the trail winds up moderately steep granite slopes to Horton Pass.

Warning: Snow often obscures this high route well into summer, so navigate carefully.

A cairn marks the top of windswept Horton Pass with its excellent views.

The side trip to the summit of Eagle Cap is outstanding and should not be missed. The summit trail begins beside a pond below the north side of Horton Pass.

Tip: It's easier to simply walk up the rocky ridge directly from the pass for about 0.4 mile to where you meet the official path.

The trail climbs steadily over rocks and snowfields, eventually switchbacking up the exposed slopes to the top. The view from here is incredible, as the rugged topography of the entire Wallowa Range spreads out in all directions. There are especially good views down the huge U-shaped gorges of East Eagle Creek and East Lostine River. To the east, Glacier Lake shimmers in its basin, and granite peaks rise in all directions. *"Wow"* pretty much sums it up.

From Horton Pass the main trail crosses meadows and semipermanent snowfields and then drops to tiny Upper Lake at the head of East Lostine Canyon. You turn right at a junction and right again just 100 yards later to reach popular Mirror Lake. On a calm morning or evening this lake lives up to its name with fine reflections of towering Eagle Cap. Continue down the trail to the east to reach deep and beautiful Moccasin Lake (excellent camps) and turn right at the junction at the lake's west end.

The trail now makes a long, strenuous climb to Glacier Pass, traveling first through forest, then meadows, and finally alpine terrain. Once again the views from the pass are terrific, but even better scenery is just ahead at Glacier Lake. On the author's personal list of Oregon's most spectacular lakes, this large alpine jewel ranks second only to incomparable Crater Lake, in the southern Cascades. When free of ice (only about two or three months out of the year), this clear pool surrounded by white granite peaks and permanent snowfields is unbelievably beautiful. Camping here is not recommended due to the fragile terrain and cold nights.

From Glacier Lake the easiest route to continue your trip is to drop by trail to Frazier Lake and then turn right and climb to Little Frazier Lake on the trail to Hawkins Pass. For hikers who don't mind some steep cross-country travel, a more scenic alternative is to cross the outlet creek of Glacier Lake and follow a boot-beaten path along the lake's east shore. Look carefully for an unmarked route that goes by a smaller upper lake, continues south over a saddle, and then drops to Prospect Lake. The stark granite basin holding this deep lake is only slightly less spectacular than the setting for Glacier Lake, and it is much more private. Unfortunately, the camps here are rocky and exposed. Reaching Little Frazier Lake requires a steep downhill scramble following the outlet creek of Prospect Lake.

Tip: In general the right (south) side of the creek provides easier going, but you'll still have to crawl around some boulders and small cliffs.

The creek itself is a joyful series of cascades and waterfalls with lots of flowers. At the bottom, go left along the north shore of Little Frazier Lake to pick up the trail.

Turn right and follow the path as it makes a moderately steep climb in several small switchbacks to Hawkins Pass.

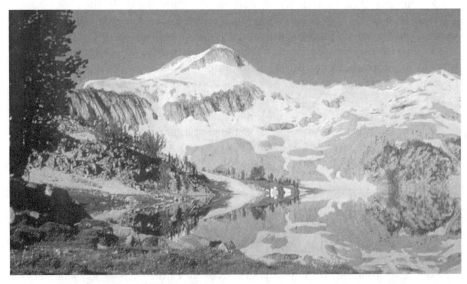

Glacier Peak over Glacier Lake

Warning: Snow remains on the north side of Hawkins Pass practically all summer.

The trail then drops into the basin at the head of the South Fork Imnaha River, which features outstanding views and acres of wildflowers. The prominent pinnacle to the southwest is Jackson Peak. There are several inviting camps both here and a bit below a lovely waterfall about 0.4 mile past where the trail crosses the stream. Farther down the canyon the views become more restricted as the forests grow thicker, but it's still a pleasant walk. Near the junction with Cliff Creek Trail, about 4.5 miles from the headwall basin, are some clearings with more nice camps.

Turn south on the Cliff Creek Trail and immediately face a chilly ford of the Imnaha River. The path then climbs steadily through forests and brushy meadows on its way up Cliff Creek. Wildflowers add color in summer, and larch trees make October equally attractive in this area. Look for deer in the meadows—and often in your camp at night. Aptly named Red Mountain towers to the east, adding to the excellent scenery. You top out at a forested pass and then turn right at a junction to reach Crater Lake, which has good camps in the trees above the north shore. Unlike most lakes in the Wallowas, this one does not fill a glacial cirque but sits in a low saddle near the pass. The lake's water level fluctuates considerably during the year. The high water of early summer is more attractive. Distant views of Krag Peak, Red Mountain, and Granite Mountain provide lovely backdrops.

Tip: If you've got an extra day, spend it on a easy flower walk to Tuck Pass and the Pine Lakes to the southeast.

To complete the loop trip, you hike west through a low saddle past a couple of shallow ponds and then make a long, fairly steep descent down the brushy avalanche slopes beside Little Kettle Creek. A seemingly endless series of switchbacks eases the grade. The trail ends at the junction with the East Eagle Trail just 0.5 mile from your car at the trailhead.

POSSIBLE ITINERARY			
	Camp	Miles	Elevation Gain
Day 1	Hidden Lake	8.8	2800
Day 2	Mirror Lake (with side trip up Eagle Cap)	12.0	3500
Day 3	Upper Imnaha Basin	10.0	2500
Day 4	Crater Lake	8.4	1500
Day 5	Out	6.7	100

CONTINUED ON PAGE 186

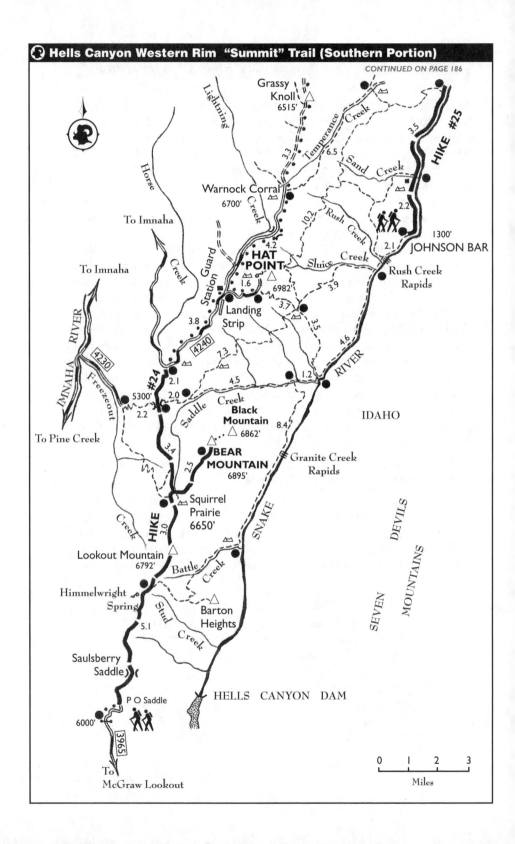

Grassy
Knoll
6515'

Lightning

Horse

Temperance

Creek

3.3

6.5

Sand

Creek

3.5

HIKE #25

Warnock Corral
6700'

To Imnaha

Creek

Guard
Station

10.2

Rush Creek

2.2

To Imnaha

Creek

4.2

HAT
POINT

1.6

6982'

Sluice

Creek

2.1

1300'

JOHNSON BAR

To Imnaha

IMNAHA RIVER

4230

Freezeout

3.8

Landing
Strip

4240

7.3

3.7

3.9

3.5

Rush Creek
Rapids

RIVER

4.6

To Pine Creek

#24

5300'

2.1

2.0

2.2

Saddle

Creek

4.5

Black
Mountain
△ 6862'

1.2

IDAHO

8.4

3.4

2.5

BEAR
MOUNTAIN
6895'

Granite Creek
Rapids

Squirrel
Prairie
6650'

SNAKE

DEVILS

HIKE

3.0

Creek

Lookout Mountain
6792'

Battle

Creek

MOUNTAINS

Himmelwright
Spring

Stud

△

Barton
Heights

SEVEN

5.1

Creek

Saulsberry
Saddle

P O Saddle

HELLS   CANYON   DAM

6000'

3965

To
McGraw Lookout

0   1   2   3

Miles

24 Hells Canyon Western Rim "Summit" Trail

RATINGS (1–10)			MILES	ELEVATION GAIN	DAYS	SHUTTLE MILEAGE
Scenery	Solitude	Difficulty				
8	8	5	53	7400	5–7	63
			(66)	(9300)	(6–9)	

MAP USFS—*Hells Canyon National Recreation Area*

USUALLY OPEN Late May to November

BEST Early to mid-June

PERMITS None

RULES Private land along Cow Creek—follow the owner's rules

CONTACT Wallowa Valley visitor center, (541) 426-4978

SPECIAL ATTRACTIONS Views; wildlife; solitude; wildflowers

PROBLEMS Limited water sources; some road walking; large burned areas; ticks

HOW TO GET THERE Reach the south starting point by driving the paved Wallowa Loop Road (Forest Road 39) for 43 miles east and south from Joseph or 28 miles north from Highway 86 at the Pine Creek junction (60 miles east of Baker City) to the well-marked Road 3965 turnoff. Drive east toward the Hells Canyon Overlook for 2.8 miles and then veer left (north) on a rough gravel road. You pass the turnoff to McGraw Lookout and continue 10.3 miles to a gate and developed trailhead.

There are two options for exiting this hike. The first is Dug Bar (see Trip 25 for directions). A slightly shorter option is to exit via Cow Creek. This route crosses private land and follows a road closed to public traffic, but hikers are allowed to walk through. This exit avoids the final steep 10 miles of the Dug Bar Road, so it is easier for those with a typical passenger car. The Cow Creek Road branches off the Dug Bar Road 0.4 mile past the bridge over Cow Creek. Park on the side so you don't block traffic.

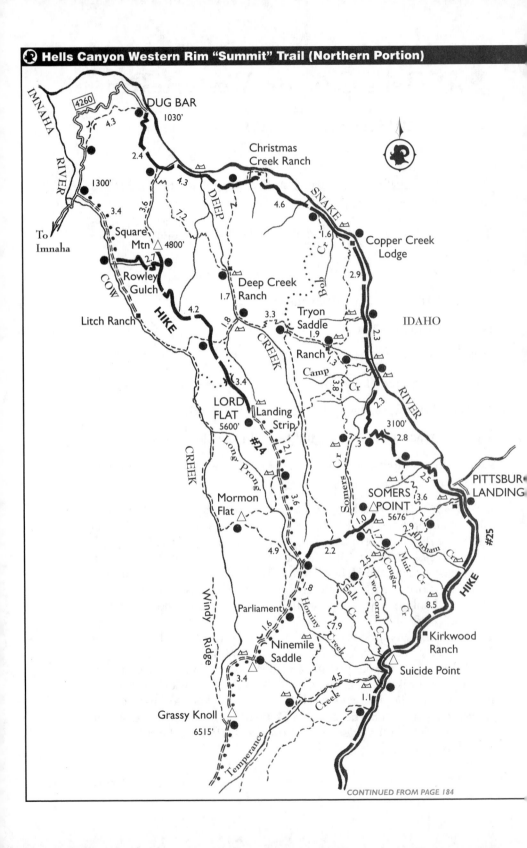

IMNAHA RIVER

4260

DUG BAR
1030'

2.4

4.3

1300'

3.6

3.4

7.2

DEEP

Square
Mtn △ 4800'

2.7

Rowley
Gulch

COW

Litch Ranch

HIKE

4.2

1.8

CREEK

Christmas
Creek Ranch

4.3

4.6

SNAKE

1.6

Bob Cr

Copper Creek
Lodge

2.9

Deep Creek
Ranch

1.7

3.3

Tryon
Saddle
1.9

Ranch
1.3

IDAHO

2.3

Camp

Cr

3.8

3.4

RIVER

2.3

LORD
FLAT
5600'

Landing
Strip

#24

2.1

3100'

2.8

CREEK

Long Prong

3.6

Mormon
Flat △

4.9

Somers Cr

.3

2.5

SOMERS
△ POINT
5676

3.6

1.0

1.7

2.9

Durham Cr

PITTSBURG
LANDING

#25

2.2

1.8

Parliament

1.6

Ninemile
Saddle

Hominy Creek

7.9

Salt Cr

Two Corral Cr

2.5

Cougar Cr

Muir Cr

8.5

HIKE

Kirkwood
Ranch

Windy Ridge

3.4

Grassy Knoll
6515'

Temperance

Creek

4.5

1.1

Suicide Point

CONTINUED FROM PAGE 184

Tip: One excellent option for avoiding the time-consuming and tedious car shuttles in Hells Canyon is to employ a shuttle service. Originally designed for rafters, these services also assist hikers by moving your vehicle between trailheads while you spend more time hiking. Fees vary and you'll have to make arrangements in advance. One such service is Hells Canyon Shuttle, (800) 785-3358.

INTRODUCTION Of the three long trails in Hells Canyon described in this guide, the Western Rim Trail is the most comfortable for backpackers. There are comparatively few steep ups and downs here since the path follows the surprisingly gentle Summit Ridge. The unbearable heat of the lower canyon is replaced by higher-elevation temperatures that are 20 or more degrees cooler. Nights too are more comfortably cool for sleeping. There is also plenty of shade among the rim's evergreen forests. On the other hand, the rim route has fewer water sources, so camping choices are limited.

Tip 1: For more solitude, hike this route before Hat Point Road opens to traffic (usually around the second week of June, but call ahead to confirm). You will have to walk over a few snowfields, but the joy of having the terrific view from Hat Point all to yourself is well worth it.

Tip 2: Don't forget to bring binoculars; wildlife is abundant.

DESCRIPTION From the south trailhead, the Western Rim Trail follows a gravel road that drops to P O Saddle.

Note: From about mid-June to mid-September this road is open to cars for the first 1.5 miles, to Saulsberry Saddle. At this point it temporarily enters the wilderness, so the Forest Service has blocked the road with a berm.

The road continues to Saulsberry Saddle, where it crosses under a set of power lines and reverts to a dirt jeep track. There are proposals to reopen this route to car traffic. While this would provide greater vehicle access to the canyon, it would also effectively ruin a terrific hike and, worse, disturb vitally important wildlife habitat. With good road access already available to the rim at Hat Point and P O Saddle, the small benefits from opening more roads would seem to be greatly outweighed by the costs.

The jeep road climbs up a wide gully to a large flat area with a mix of forests and meadows.

Tip: Two springs can be found to the west of the trail for those in need of water.

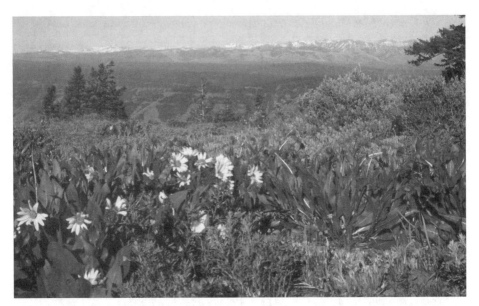

Himmelwright Meadow

The route continues northeast along the ridge and then breaks out of the trees at the expansive meadows near Himmelwright Spring. In June this meadow is a flower bonanza, choked with the large white blossoms of wyethia as well as yellow balsamroot and a smattering of other species. Views extend to the snowy peaks of the distant Wallowa Mountains. Unfortunately, cows are allowed to trample the whole area, so the trail can be smelly and muddy, and camping is problematic.

After descending from Himmelwright Meadow, the old jeep road climbs a bit and then comes to a junction with the Battle Creek Trail. This route veers off to the right on its way down to the Snake River. Continuing north, your trail makes a gradual ascent, sometimes in a tunnel of trees, to Lookout Mountain. Views are partly obstructed by trees, but the open area on top supports a wealth of wildflowers.

The old road pretty much ends at Lookout Mountain, although a jeep track continues as far as Squirrel Prairie. You drop a bit to Benjamin Spring, which may run dry by mid to late summer, and continue the moderate descent to a junction. To the left is the trail to Marks Cabin and a spring. The Western Rim Trail goes right and drops to the sloping meadow and the (usually) year-round creek in Squirrel Prairie. This is an excellent place to camp, although the presence of a healthy bear population makes it prudent to hang your food. (So far, the bears in Hells Canyon have not presented a problem for campers. Proper food storage will help keep it that way.)

Tip: A superb side trip from here follows the Bear Mountain Trail east through meadows and a forest of burned snags. The trail climbs a bit and then follows a wide ridge all the way to the outstanding view atop Bear Mountain. The perspective of the snowy Seven Devils Mountains, appearing deceptively close across the gaping chasm, is particularly noteworthy.

Back on the Western Rim Trail, the route soon becomes a footpath, but travel remains easy, with only modest ups and downs. More snags and regrowing trees provide further evidence of old fires. Views alternate between the Freezeout and Imnaha canyons to the west and Hells Canyon and the peaks in Idaho to the east. You may even spot the lookout tower on Hat Point in the distance to the north. About 3.7 miles from Squirrel Prairie is Freezeout Saddle, where the Bench and Saddle Creek trails cross our route.

The Western Rim Trail goes straight and makes a well-graded climb up a rocky ridge covered with wildflowers, bunchgrass, and a few evergreens. Excellent views provide interest and variety as the trail shifts from one side of the ridge to the other. A little before the final switchbacks are two (usually flowing) creeklets.

Tip: Stock up on water here since this is the last opportunity for several miles.

At the top of the climb is the gravel Hat Point Road (Forest Road 4240), which serves as the trail for the next several miles. If your trip is in early June, the road walk should be pleasantly quiet, otherwise you must share the route with cars.

Turn right on the road and soon reach walk-in Saddle Creek Campground. Here there are picnic tables, campsites, and breathtaking views, but no water. The road makes a series of ups and downs through subalpine-fir forests and recently burned areas as it tours the top of the ridge overlooking Hells Canyon. Several viewpoints along the way will keep your camera busy. The road eventually works away from the ridge, passes some buildings beside the Memaloose helitack and airstrip, and reaches the junction with Road 315 to Hat Point. This entire area (and for many miles to come) was burned by the Summit Fire in 1989, which left behind a seemingly endless silver ghost forest that is interesting but provides little shade and is rather monotonous. Small lodgepole pines have sprouted a new forest, but they are still fairly short and unimpressive.

The quickest way to continue the Western Rim Trail is to go straight on the road toward Warnock Corral, but to come this far and skip visiting Hat Point would be absurd. So turn right and make the moderate 1.7-mile climb up the road to the Hat Point Lookout. This 90-foot tower

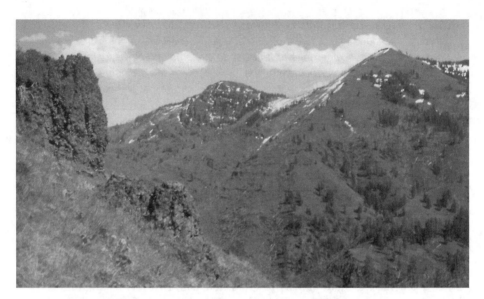

Bear and Black mountains from near Freezeout Saddle

is staffed in summer, and the person assigned here enjoys views that defy description. The look down to the Snake River, flowing over a vertical mile below, is amazing. Even more thrilling, however, are the seemingly endless vistas of canyon slopes, the mountains in Idaho, and the distant Wallowa Mountains in Oregon. In early July the meadows provide gorgeous foregrounds with a colorful array of wildflowers. A picnic area and a short interpretive trail surround the lookout, providing information as well as scenic lunch spots.

> **Tip:** To spend the night at Hat Point, continue north another 0.3 mile to Sacajawea Campground with its year-round spring.

To continue on the Western Rim Trail, return to Road 4240 and turn right. The road immediately passes the Memaloose Guard Station, then slowly descends beside the headwaters of Lightning Creek. At a gate, the road changes from gravel to dirt and then continues down to a nice view from Sluice Creek Saddle before climbing a bit to the Warnock Corral Trailhead in a small meadow. Camping here is pleasant (especially before the road is open) with a spring and small creek for water and a few green trees providing shade amidst the burned snags of the ghost forest. The Temperance Creek Trail drops to the northeast from here on its way to the Snake River.

From Warnock Corral the Western Rim Trail follows a recently reopened four-wheel-drive road that winds north through more of the extensive burn area from the 1989 fire. Although reopened by congressional mandate, the need for this jeep road is debatable at best. For now it is used primarily by hunters in the fall, so early-summer hikers should have it all to themselves. There is neither water nor shade on this rather dull segment, so it can get surprisingly hot for this elevation. The road/trail passes a marked side route to Sleepy Ridge and, 0.5 mile later, finally leaves the ghost forest and enters more attractive terrain. You keep straight at the junction with a jeep road to Windy Ridge and then climb briefly to the view atop aptly named Grassy Knoll.

From this high point the route cuts through a nearly pure stand of even-age lodgepole pines (the legacy of a fire several decades ago) for 2 miles to a fence line. Beyond this the terrain becomes more diverse and interesting, with better views but also several steep ups and downs—a rarity for this hike. After about 1 mile is a low point called Indian Grave Saddle, where there are an excellent camp and a spring with a pipe and horse trough. Refill your water bottles here. The road now enters a more recent burn area and makes a quick climb to a ridge.

Tip: A worthwhile side trip goes south from here to an unnamed open knoll with terrific views.

The Western Rim Trail goes north along the rim before dropping to Ninemile Saddle (more views). Shortly beyond the next hill is an unmarked jeep trail to the west that goes 0.2 mile to a spring and an old cabin (possible camps here).

Atop the next hill is a junction and a large meadow area identified on maps as "Parliament." No other legislature on the planet could possibly have enjoyed a better view! To the east drops the enormous gorge of Hells Canyon, while to the west is a gentler slope of forests that drop off into the canyons and ridges of Imnaha River country. Elk were the only legislators present during the author's visit. Leaving "Capitol Hill," so to speak, the road remains easy walking as it gradually descends past viewpoints for 1.8 miles to a junction.

Veering off to the right is the highly recommended up and down route to Somers Point. Views along this path—especially the jaw-dropper from Somers Point itself—are among the most memorable on this trip. The first 200 yards follow a jeep road, but the route soon becomes a pleasant footpath. The trail passes some nice camps in a saddle after 1.1 miles. You keep right at a junction just west of an unobtrusive radio tower and then descend through attractive forests. The last mile to Somers Point is over a wide and spectacular meadowy ridge with lots of views and wildflowers.

The view you'll enjoy from the end of Somers Point is outstanding. The river can be seen in two different directions, contorted canyon

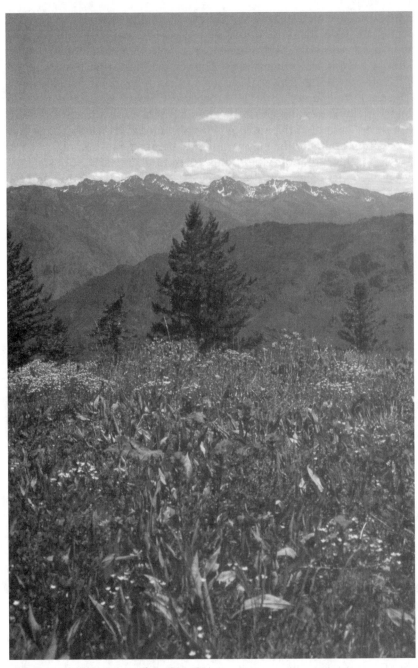

Seven Devils Mountains from Hat Point

walls stretch for miles, and the snowy peaks of Idaho provide a fine backdrop. Pittsburg Landing, with its boat ramp and campground, is directly below on the Idaho side of the river. Fires in 1996 left some snags but these can't diminish the scene.

Tip: Binoculars will come in handy to spot wildlife and rafters.

A view like this is hard to leave and, fortunately, there is an inviting camp nearby. A spring with pipe and horse trough is 200 yards north of and below the trail 0.2 mile west of Somers Point. Excellent camps are found another 200 yards west of the spring in a strip of trees.

Warning: If you leave camp, be sure to hang your food first. When the author returned from his own evening stroll, a curious young bear was busy trying to push over the tent. No harm was done, but consider yourself on notice.

Back at the Somers Point junction, the Western Rim Trail continues to follow the road on its gentle course to the north. After curving left, the route heads back toward the ridge but generally remains in the trees. After making a long, fairly gradual descent, the road starts to break out into more open country. A short side trail goes left near here to Dorrance Cow Camp, where there are a cabin and some good camps. The main trail continues north over a grassy hill and drops through view-packed bunchgrass meadows to the south end of the Lord Flat landing strip. Despite its remote location, this airstrip's grassy 2000-foot "tarmac" gets a surprising amount of use by Forest Service personnel, hunters, and others. Water is also available here.

From the strip the Western Rim Trail veers left on a jeep track and gradually drops down open slopes. Look for wildlife such as elk and black bears here. The jeep road finally ends near a tiny pond, after which the trail descends 19 switchbacks as it closely follows the Summit Ridge. To your immediate right is Deep Creek Canyon, while to the left is Cow Creek's rugged defile. Your route switchbacks down to a saddle and a junction with sketchy use paths heading both left and right. Continue straight and trace an up-and-down route along the ridge for about 2 miles to Fingerboard Saddle.

A good trail crosses our route here providing a possible exit to the Cow Creek Road. This is the shortest way out for hikers in a hurry. To exit from here, turn left, drop to Cow Creek, and follow the road downstream through Litch Ranch and out to your car.

If you decide to stick with the Western Rim Trail, keep straight from Fingerboard Saddle and follow a rollercoaster route along the ridge. The north end of Summit Ridge is much narrower and more rugged than the south end, but it also has more continuous views and

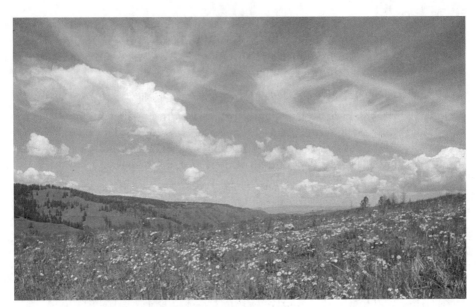

Meadows near Somers Point

fewer trees. The trail is often indistinct, but since it closely follows the ridgeline you shouldn't get lost.

Warning: Water along the ridge is scarce to nonexistent—carry extra.

Loop around the headwaters of Little Deep Creek to the east and make a sometimes-steep descent from a highpoint on the ridge to a saddle. The trail goes over another hill before facing the final short climb to Square Mountain. The Rowley Gulch Trail goes left and makes a steep switchbacking descent from the saddle just south of Square Mountain. Having come this far, however, you really should make the climb to Square Mountain to enjoy its views all the way to the Snake River near Dug Bar.

If Dug Bar is your chosen exit, follow the Western Rim Trail north from Square Mountain as it follows Dug Creek through a mix of forests and meadows to a junction first with the Bench Trail and then with the Snake River Trail (beware of poison ivy near here). The trail goes over a small rise with excellent views down to Dug Bar Ranch and drops down to the river-level trailhead.

To exit via Rowley Gulch, the steep route (often easy to lose) switchbacks down a ridge and then goes over to a side canyon before paralleling the seasonal creek in Rowley Gulch to Cow Creek Road. Turn right and follow this road through attractive, mostly open country usually well above the stream back to your car.

Note: *Please be respectful of the private land here by keeping gates open or closed as you found them and by not camping.*

Note: *The three trips described in Hells Canyon (24–26) are all one-way, point-to-point hikes. For those unable to arrange a car shuttle, it is also possible to devise several long and spectacular loop trips in the canyon. One of the best begins at Dug Bar, goes up the Snake River Trail to Somers Creek, and then returns to Dug Bar via the Bench Trail over Tryon Saddle. This trip is a total of 42 miles and is at its best in early to mid-May. A second trip, which peaks in early June—although with some snow at the highest elevations, begins at the Freezeout Trailhead and follows the Bench Trail to Kneeland Place. The route then climbs steeply to Somers Point and returns to the Freezeout Trailhead via the Western Rim Trail. The total distance for this loop is 58 miles. With some creativity and a good map, many other loop trips of various lengths can be planned.*

Warnings: *Less-used connecting trails are often faint and difficult to find on the ground. Also, the canyon's great changes in elevation create radically different environments. Hence, while one part of your planned loop is cool, green, and beautiful, a lower part of the same trip may be hot, dry, and brown. Prepare accordingly.*

POSSIBLE ITINERARY

	Camp	Miles	Elevation Gain
Day 1	Squirrel Prairie (with side trip to Bear Mountain)	13.1	2200
Day 2	Sacajawea Campground (Hat Point)	11.4	2300
Day 3	Indian Grave Saddle	12.2	1100
Day 4	Somers Point	6.6	1200
Day 5	Lord Flat	8.9	1000
Day 6	Out	13.7	1500

RATINGS (1–10)			MILES	ELEVATION GAIN	DAYS	SHUTTLE MILEAGE
Scenery	Solitude	Difficulty				
10	7	8	41	6000	4–5	N/A

MAP USFS—*Hells Canyon National Recreation Area*

USUALLY OPEN All year

BEST Mid-April to early May

PERMITS None

RULES No fires within 0.25 mile of the Snake River

CONTACT Wallowa Valley visitor center, (541) 426-4978

SPECIAL ATTRACTIONS Whitewater rafters to watch; historic sites; wildlife; great canyon scenery

PROBLEMS Complicated and expensive boat transportation; rattlesnakes, ticks, and black widow spiders (especially in the spring and early summer); no shade—it can be extremely hot; lots of poison ivy

> *Note:* See maps for Trip 24 (pages 184 and 186).

HOW TO GET THERE The logistics of starting this hike are unusually complicated. A very long and tedious car shuttle from Hells Canyon Dam to Dug Bar is one option. This would allow you to enjoy the trail's entire length, but it also would require making arrangements for a short boat ride downstream to Battle Creek, where Oregon's river trail starts. A second option (with a much shorter car shuttle) is to start the trip from the Freezeout Trailhead (see Trip 26). This requires a climb over Freezeout Saddle, where there is likely to be some snow through April. The route then descends the Saddle Creek Trail to reach the Snake River Trail about 8 miles downstream from Battle Creek.

> *Warning:* The Saddle Creek Trail includes several stream crossings that in the spring can be cold and rather treacherous.

Still another plan (and the one recommended here) necessitates only one car, but you must make arrangements at least two weeks in advance with a jet-boat operator to pick you up at Dug Bar and drop you off upstream. The larger companies are happy to help, but you'll have to work around their regular tour schedules. As of 2006, expect to pay between $60 and $120 for boat transport from Dug Bar to about Johnson Bar. A final option, which avoids bad roads altogether, is to leave your car in Lewiston, Idaho, take the jet boat upstream to your chosen drop off, and then arrange for the boat to pick you up for the ride back down to Lewiston at the end of the hike. This option requires that you stick with a set schedule on the trail to make the prearranged pickup time, and you'll probably have to pay for two boat trips.

Tip: See the note in Trip 24 concerning car-shuttle services for hikes in Hells Canyon.

Note: While jet boats are recommended here as the most convenient transportation for backpackers, they are not necessary for this hike. Many environmentalists believe these boats should be restricted or even prohibited from using the river to reduce noise, fumes, and beach erosion. If you are morally opposed to the use of jet boats, do not avoid this outstanding trip as a result. Use one of the other options noted above. The trip may even be improved by being more of a wilderness experience. Ultimately, the best solution is for the Forest Service to fulfill the Snake River Trail's enormous potential by completing the final 5-mile segment from Hells Canyon Dam to Battle Creek. The initial investment would be repaid many times over by producing one of the continent's grandest long hikes and helping local tourism.

To reach the Dug Bar Trailhead, drive north from the tiny community of Imnaha on a paved county road. Beyond Fence Creek Ranch the road changes to dirt and becomes steep, narrow, and winding. The drive is long and sometimes rough but incredibly scenic. It ends at Dug Bar, 30 tiring miles from Imnaha.

Warning: The last 8 miles are especially steep and difficult. When the road is wet, a four-wheel-drive vehicle is highly recommended.

INTRODUCTION Two words sum up the experience of hiking Oregon's Snake River Trail—"spectacular" and "exhausting." With all due respect to the marvelous canyon scenery found along the Rogue River, the Owyhee River, and many other Oregon streams, they all pale in comparison to the enormity of Hells Canyon. The Snake River Trail provides perhaps the ultimate backpacking experience in the canyon. Only the most jaded traveler will fail to return with nothing more than a sore neck from so much time spent looking up to the canyon's rim thousands of feet above. More serious threats than a sore neck, however, are rattlesnakes and poison ivy, so you must spend at least as much time looking down as up.

*Two **Tips** for those looking to tackle this major adventure:*

1) Summer days are blisteringly hot and nights uncomfortably warm. Dress accordingly and be prepared to sleep on top of your bag.

2) In many places poison ivy is so abundant you simply cannot avoid the stuff. Try using one of those shielding products you apply before contact and/or special soaps to wash off the toxins afterward. People who are particularly allergic should probably avoid this hike altogether.

DESCRIPTION Pick up your prearranged boat ride at Dug Bar and plan on a long, exciting, and informative trip upriver to the recommended drop off opposite Johnson Bar. The larger companies typically stop on the way up at Kirkwood Ranch, an interesting museum that is well worth a visit. It will be early afternoon by the time you disembark. You must scramble up the bank a bit to reach the trail.

Tip: Before starting the downstream trek consider a short exploration upstream. Rush Creek Rapids is a good nearby goal and logical turnaround point.

Downstream from Johnson Bar, the wildly scenic route stays close to the river and soon comes to a fine camp at (probably dry) Yreka Creek—obtain water from the Snake River. The path then crosses a huge rock shelf called Eagle's Nest, where the trail has been blasted into the side of the rock. Take a moment to marvel at the work involved—not to mention the quantity of dynamite it must have taken. This path was built in the 1930s by Civilian Conservaton Corps workers, who did an admirable job. About 2.2 miles from the takeout point is the Sand Creek game warden's cabin. Further downstream, at Alum Bar Rapids, the Idaho side boasts a colorful area of exposed yellow cliffs.

The trail works around a bend in the river and then tours a grassy bench above the stream. You pass a marked junction with a very sketchy "trail" up Dry Gulch and then go around a large, fenced meadowy flat. In a confusing section near the north end of this pasture, the trail crosses the fence and goes down to Temperance Creek Ranch. You make a bridged crossing of Temperance Creek and come immediately to a junction in the trees. You can camp upstream amid this creek's lush riparian vegetation.

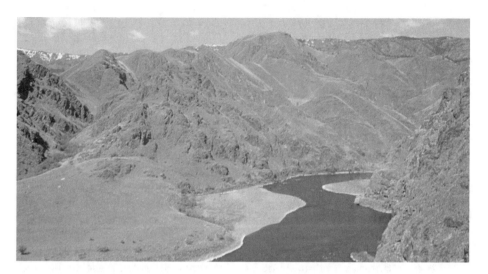

View below Suicide Point

Now the Snake River Trail goes north, passes the massive cliffs of Suicide Point (across the river in Idaho), and reaches good camps and a cabin at the flats of Salt Creek.

Tip: *A possible side trip climbs the steep Salt Creek Trail to a series of excellent viewpoints above the river.*

Continuing on the Snake River Trail, cross Two Corral Creek, briefly follow close to the river, then go across a large, sloping bench. Near the north end of this bench is Slaughter Gulch (often dry). The trail now drops to the riverside and hugs the shore beside steep cliffs. The route is chiseled into the canyon walls and, despite staying close to river level, is constantly making tiny ups and downs. At the crossing of Cougar Creek there are good views across the river to the meadowy flat holding Kirkwood Ranch.

The rugged trail continues to hug the cliffs on the Oregon side for the next mile or two before breaking out onto a meadowy bench across from Idaho's Kirby Bar. At Muir Creek are water and some possible spots to eat lunch or camp. The alternating pattern of steep slopes and river benches continues as you cross a set of cliffs and reach the bench at Durham Creek (more potential camps). For the next 2 miles the trail goes through a narrow section of the canyon where both the Oregon and Idaho trails have been carved out of the hillsides and cliffs. You are likely to see far more people on the Idaho side's trail since that popular route has easy access for dayhikers from Pittsburg Landing.

Landmarks are mainly on the opposite shore and include the trailhead at Upper Pittsburg Landing and, later, the car campground at Lower Pittsburg. On the Oregon side, the trail crosses an arid bench to a junction with a steep path going up Robertson Gulch and then continues to the Pittsburg Guard Station.

In the miles ahead the Snake River cuts through a particularly narrow and steep-walled part of Hells Canyon. To avoid this difficult section, you are forced to make a long, sometimes rugged, but highly scenic detour. First your path climbs inland to the Bench Trail, some 1500 feet above. The climb is steep in places and, as is true on the entire trail, exposed to the sun. Start with full water bottles and carry your own shade—a hat. The route contours away from Pittsburg and climbs up a draw to a point about 500 feet above the river. Near the head of this draw is a spring with possible water. The trail then traces an up-and-down course for about 1 mile to the crossing of Pleasant Valley Creek, with water and some shade. Now the climb really gets under way as the rocky path leads up a small ridge, gaining a little over 1000 feet in 1 mile. Just short of the high point is a junction with the Bench Trail in a large meadow with terrific views up to Somers Point.

The two trails follow the same route north for the next 2.8 miles. After 1.5 beautiful ridge-and-meadow miles the fun abruptly ends as the trail steeply climbs a shadeless gully to a pass. Take a well-deserved rest at the top to enjoy the great views in all directions. As the trail descends toward Somers Creek there are some fine views down to the river.

At a junction near the rounded summit called Englishman Hill, the Bench Trail goes left a short distance to Somers Creek (good camps), while the Snake River Trail turns right and continues its descent back to the river. After you make a couple of quick switchbacks, the often steep route follows a tributary canyon of Somers Creek down to the main stream. A pleasant riparian zone of dense deciduous vegetation and a few ponderosa pines hosts the trail as it parallels the rushing stream. The route requires three creek crossings that may get your feet wet but aren't difficult.

Warning: Be particularly alert for poison ivy and rattlesnakes through this section.

Where you return to the Snake River there are good campsites near an old cabin. At Camp Creek, a short distance farther north, are more

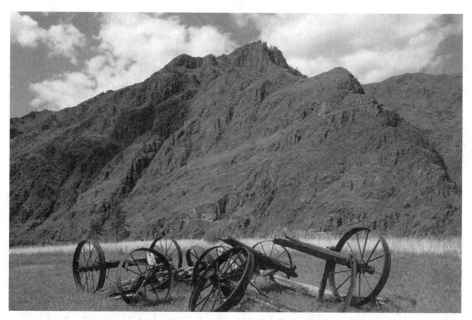

Farm equipment relics at Kirkwood Ranch

camps and a junction with a trail that climbs back up to the Bench Trail near Tryon Creek Ranch.

To continue your tour, closely follow the banks of the Snake River as it cuts a surprisingly straight path north for the next few miles. Steep cliffs on both sides of the canyon provide exciting scenery. The Idaho side no longer has a trail, as that path's northern terminus was Pittsburg Landing. About 0.4 mile north of Camp Creek is Tryon Creek, where there is a good camp and you will have a chance to refill your water bottles. If this spot doesn't suit you, there are more camps at Lookout Creek just over 1 mile farther north. After Lookout Creek the trail passes along the base of some impressive cliffs, and in places has been blasted right into the side of them.

After a junction with a sketchy trail just before Lonepine Creek (usually dry), your trail leads well above the raging Snake River as it cuts through a particularly narrow segment of the canyon. Near Highrange Rapids is an old mine shaft, just above the trail, that is protected as a nursery for bats. The trail then works back down to river level and returns to its pattern of miniature ups and downs blasted into the cliffs.

Just past a second mine tunnel, the trail splits. The official trail climbs to the left, while to the right are a boat landing and the lush oasis of Copper Creek Lodge. This modern facility is run by a commercial boat operator. In fact, you may have stopped here on the boat ride up. It includes several modern cabins, manicured lawns and shade trees, running water, gift items and souvenirs, and dining facilities. Hikers need reservations to spend the night or eat here; call (800) 522-6966. The trails near here are used by dayhikers from Copper Creek Lodge, so this is one of the few areas where you can expect company on this trip.

Shortly beyond the lodge you cross a wide bench where there is a junction near Bob Creek.

Tip: *Shortly after crossing this creek, look for a short spur trail that goes upstream to a small waterfall.*

Several trees on the flat meadow area near Bob Creek make this a particularly good campsite. As you leave the dayhikers behind, the Snake River Trail remains close to the river until Cat Creek, where it detours around an abandoned ranch. A sketchy trail ascends the slopes south of here on its way to Tryon Saddle.

To continue your tour, traverse a large meadowy bench above Roland Bar Rapids and then arrive at Roland Creek. This small creek usually flows all year so stock up on water here. For the next several miles the Snake River Trail travels a rugged up-and-down course well away from the river over terrain that will keep your heart pounding, from both the exertion and the views.

Tip: *Elk are common. Keep an eye out for wildlife.*

The detour away from the river starts with a sometimes steep and rocky 600-foot climb from Roland Creek to a saddle. The trail then follows a less strenuous up-and-down course to the buildings of abandoned Dorrance Ranch. Just past the ranch the trail splits. To the right, a path drops back down to the Snake River and then continues to Christmas Creek Ranch. The official Snake River Trail keeps left, crosses Bean Creek (usually flowing), and then drops a bit around a ridge to Christmas Creek. Shortly beyond this small stream is the junction with the return loop of the trail to Christmas Creek Ranch. Next is yet another climb, although this time at a fairly moderate grade, up a view-packed slope to a junction with the spectacular path to Deep Creek Ranch.

Tip: *If you have an extra day, this trail is well worth taking as a long side trip.*

After crossing Thorn Spring Creek near an old cabin, the trail climbs a bit more and then begins the steep 1100-foot descent back to the Snake River.

The trail returns to the river just above Deep Creek Bar. There is plenty of water here, as well as a collection of interesting shacks and old machinery from Chinese miners. Several luxurious camps in the vicinity cater to whitewater rafters and feature such amenities as picnic tables and an outhouse.

Warning: You must ford Deep Creek here—which can be a bit tricky in the spring—so use caution.

To complete your adventure, continue along the Snake River another 1.1 miles to Dug Creek. You turn up this side stream and travel through the dense grasses and vegetation along the creek.

Warning: The stinging nettles and poison ivy in this section are so thick they are impossible to avoid.

Flood damage has made the trail easy to lose as it crosses and recrosses the creek. Often the easiest alternative is to simply walk up the streambed itself. After about 0.8 mile the trail finally works away from the creek (although the poison ivy remains in force) and reaches a junction. Turn right and climb a bit to reach a great view overlooking Dug Bar and then drop steeply to the ranch. The public trail is well marked and goes to the right around the ranch area.

Tip: Don't miss the short side trail to a sign discussing the Nez Perce Indians' crossing of the Snake River near this location in 1877. The courageous band of Native Americans led by Chief Joseph traveled through here on a heroic (and ultimately futile) journey in search of freedom.

From here it is only a few hundred yards to the parking area near the boat ramp at the trailhead.

POSSIBLE ITINERARY			
	Camp	Miles	Elevation Gain
Day 1	Temperance Creek	6.8	500
Day 2	Pittsburg	8.5	500
Day 3	Bob Creek	13.2	2600
Day 4	Out	12.5	2400

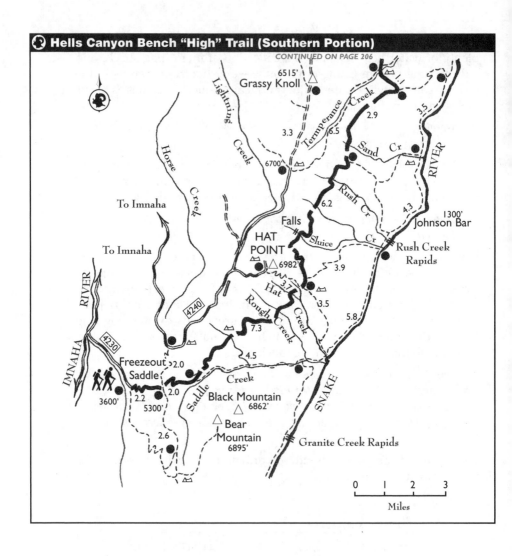

CONTINUED ON PAGE 206

6515'
Grassy Knoll

Lightning Creek

Horse Creek

Temperance Creek

3.3

6.5

2.9

1.1

3.5

6700'

Sand Cr

RIVER

Rush Cr

6.2

4.3

1300'
Johnson Bar

To Imnaha

To Imnaha

Falls

HAT
POINT

6982'

Sluice

Cr

Rush Creek
Rapids

3.9

3.7

3.5

Hat

Rough Creek

Creek

5.8

4240

7.3

4.5

SNAKE

IMNAHA RIVER

4230

Freezeout
Saddle

2.0

Creek

Saddle Creek

3600'

2.2

2.0

Black Mountain
6862'

5300'

Bear
Mountain
6895'

2.6

Granite Creek Rapids

0   1   2   3

Miles

Hells Canyon Bench "High" Trail

RATINGS (1–10)			MILES	ELEVATION GAIN	DAYS	SHUTTLE MILEAGE
Scenery	Solitude	Difficulty				
10	8	8	63	14,900	5–8	46

MAP   USFS—*Hells Canyon National Recreation Area*

USUALLY OPEN   April to November

BEST   Early to mid-May

PERMITS   None

RULES   No fires within 0.25 mile of Snake River

CONTACT   Wallowa Valley visitor center, (541) 426-4978

SPECIAL ATTRACTIONS   Views; abundant wildlife; wildflowers; solitude

PROBLEMS   Rattlesnakes; poor road access; poison ivy; often very hot; rough trail; several burn areas; ticks (especially in the spring)

HOW TO GET THERE   To reach the north trailhead of this hike, drive to the end of the Dug Bar Road (see Trip 25 description). The south trailhead is located south of Imnaha. Take the county road along the east bank of the Imnaha River for 13 miles. Shortly before a bridge, turn left on Forest Road 4230 (marked SADDLE CREEK TRAIL). Keep left at the first fork and continue for 3 miles to the Freezeout Trailhead at the roadend.

> *Tip:* See the note in Trip 24 concerning car-shuttle services for hikes in Hells Canyon.

INTRODUCTION   For lovers of canyon scenery and wildflowers, the Bench Trail through Hells Canyon is the experience of a lifetime. Following a mid-canyon route about halfway between the river and the Summit Ridge, this spectacular tour provides a greater variety of scenery than any other long trail in the canyon. Not only are there views across the canyon to the peaks in Idaho, but also down into the

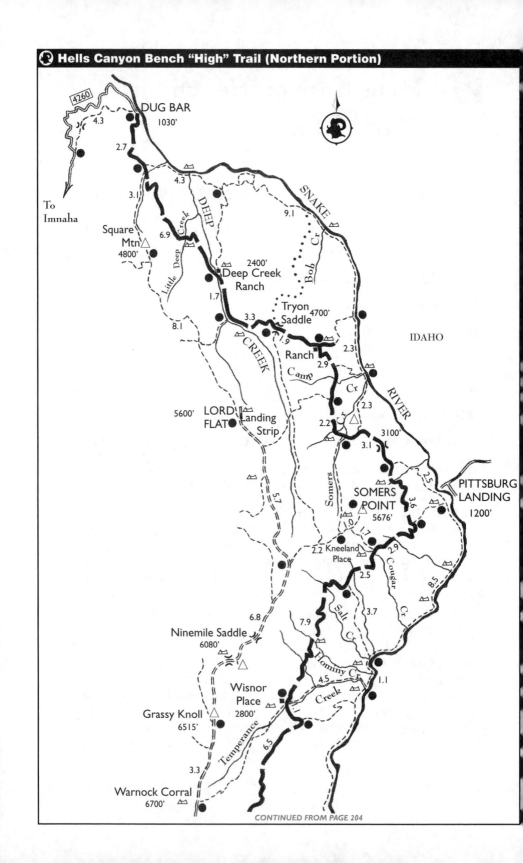

CONTINUED FROM PAGE 204

depths below, up to the contorted canyon walls above, and, often most impressive of all, of the scenic meadows right at the hiker's feet. Photographers must become very choosy to avoid running out of film (or card memory). This trail also travels through the finest examples of native bunchgrass in Oregon—a plant community lost elsewhere to the hooves of cattle and introduced plant species. In season, wildflowers and wildlife are perhaps more abundant here than on any other long trail in the state.

Despite the awesome scenery, hikers rarely travel this route, since the great distances and rugged terrain keep out all but the best-conditioned backpackers. Horse packers are much more common, although even they are rather few and far between. You'll probably have most of this wonderful hike all to yourself.

Note: Trail signs usually identify this as the HIGH TRAIL. Users, however, more often refer to it as the Bench Trail, since this is a better description of the terrain.

Warnings: Those who choose to come here must be prepared for the rigors of this place. The second half of this hike is particularly rugged, with numerous steep climbs and descents over sun-baked slopes. (Fortunately, unlike on the Snake River Trail, there are usually enough trees to provide shade at rest stops.) At lower elevations you may encounter poison ivy. Rattlesnakes inhabit the entire length of the trail. Temperatures, while more comfortable than at the bottom of the canyon, can be very hot on sunny afternoons. In a few places the route is easy to lose where game and livestock trails veer off in all directions and grasses obscure the path—good route finding instincts will come in handy.

Tip: Fans of watching wildlife should carry binoculars. Use them in the early morning and evening to scan the grassy slopes and rock ledges. There is a good chance of spotting elk, deer, bighorn sheep, black bears, coyotes, and maybe even a mountain lion. As you sit quietly and continue to search, more animals seem inevitably to come into view. It's great fun!

DESCRIPTION Your route begins with a long series of moderately steep switchbacks up a grassy slope to Freezeout Saddle. (Odds are very good you will be hot and sweaty after the 1700-foot climb, and "freezing" will be the last thing on your mind.) In many ways Freezeout Saddle is the focal point of hiking in Hells Canyon. In addition to the Bench Trail, the Western Rim Trail (see Trip 24) cuts through here on its way south to McGraw Lookout and north to Hat Point, and there is access to the Snake River via the Saddle Creek Trail. Finally, this is one of the few locations in the canyon with reasonable access for dayhikers to such landmarks as Bear Mountain.

To hike the Bench Trail, go straight from the saddle and descend a mostly open slope with several exceptional views of smooth-sided Bear Mountain and craggy Black Mountain to the south. The trail passes through a large burn area—the first of many on this trip—whose snags provide habitat for a large population of Lewis' and other woodpeckers. After 2 miles is a junction with the Saddle Creek Trail where you turn left.

As the Bench Trail goes north, several patterns that will hold true for most of this trip soon become apparent. For the most part, the trail is gently graded, following the canyon slopes at elevations between 3500 and 4500 feet. To allow this, it contours out across the ridges and into the creek canyons in a seemingly endless series of zigzags. Large meadowy benches sometimes provide a platform for the trail, but the "in-out" pattern predominates. The river, flowing some 3000 feet below, is rarely visible. Another interesting pattern is provided by the vegetation. On the north-facing slopes are surprisingly lush forests of Douglas fir and ponderosa pine, along with numerous shrubs and ground-cover plants. On drier, south-facing slopes only the occasional ponderosa pine survives amidst rocky meadows sprinkled with wildflowers. The meadowy benches and ridges are perhaps most scenic of all, with breathtaking views and thousands of flowers. Look for balsamroot, lupine, phlox, wallflower, yarrow, paintbrush, lomatium, gilia, brodiaea, and countless others.

With these patterns in place, your route begins with a long, undulating approach to a prominent ridge about 5 miles northeast. The trail has only moderate ups and downs, and numerous small creeks provide water, so the hiking is easy and enjoyable. At Log Creek are the first good campsites. Upon finally reaching the ridge, you are rewarded with a large grassy area and excellent views of the cliffs above. Shortly beyond the ridge, the route crosses Rough Creek above a small falls and then continues through forest to crossings of the several branches of Hat Creek.

About 100 feet after the last branch of Hat Creek is a sheepherder's cabin on the right, and just beyond is a junction with the trail from Hat Point. The cabin is usually open and is a good shelter if it rains.

Warning: There are lots of mice in this cabin. Hang your food and be prepared for a long night of listening to the sounds of scurrying rodents.

Keep straight at the junction with the Hat Point Trail and drop another 100 yards to a second junction, this one with a trail to the right that goes past a corral on a grassy bench before descending to the Snake River.

Now the Bench Trail goes north for 0.2 mile to yet another junction. You turn left and immediately enjoy terrific views of the impressive cliffs below Hat Point—still sporting plenty of snow in early May.

Sticking with the Bench Trail, the route traces a surprisingly gentle course as it circles the headwaters of Sluice Creek. Towering above are the awesome cliffs and rock pinnacles of Hat Point. At the final branch of Sluice Creek the route passes below an impressive waterfall—the best on the entire trip. The trail then continues to crossings of Rattlesnake Creek (a reminder to keep an eye out for these creatures), and Rush Creek. A little beyond Rush Creek is the simple gravesite of Charlie Gordon (1901–1918) for whom there is no epitaph, but the years indicate he died far too young. A little further along is a junction with a faint trail to Sand Creek and the Snake River.

Continuing north, the rambling route passes through scattered burn areas as it gradually gains elevation and works toward the top of the rugged divide separating Temperance Creek from the main canyon. The trail reaches the top of this wide and very beautiful meadowy ridge and then follows it for about 1 mile. You pass a fenced corral and then go around the right side of a grassy knoll to a saddle with a junction. Turn left and descend very steeply on a rocky trail (watch your step), losing 1200 feet to a ford of Temperance Creek. The old Wisnor Place homestead is on the opposite bank. There are excellent camps here— some of the best along the entire trail.

The Temperance Creek Trail meets the Bench Trail here. Flood damage in 1996 closed much of this trail, so it may be hard to see on the ground. To continue your tour, keep right and contour for 0.2 mile to a crossing of Bull Creek (more camps). The trail then makes a series of ups and downs as it traverses open, grassy ridges and canyons. After crossing Cove Creek (beware of poison ivy) the trail makes a determined assault up a side canyon on its way to Hominy Saddle, almost 1000 feet above. From the saddle the trail turns left and follows a fence-line up the ridge before dropping to Hominy Creek (good camps).

Returning to its familiar "into canyon-out ridge" course, the 8-mile tour between Hominy Creek and Kneeland Place is easy, mostly level hiking over open, view-packed slopes. The only problem may be losing the sometimes overgrown path as your attention is turned to the view rather than the trail. The Salt Creek Trail intersects your route at one of the many meadowy ridges. Watch for elk in this area. Cross Two Buck

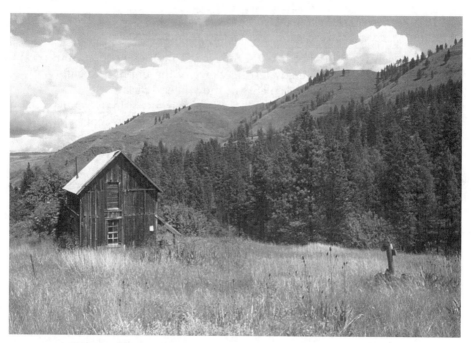

Wisnor Place

Creek and continue to Cougar Creek at the site of the old Kneeland Place (long gone). Lots of ponderosa pines and riparian shrubs make this a choice campsite—although horse packers seem to think so too, so you may be crowded out.

Tip 1: *The best camps are about 200 yards upstream near a spring.*

Tip 2: *An excellent but steep side trip from here climbs to the outstanding view at Somers Point, although this high ridge may still have some snow in May.*

Not far beyond the Kneeland Place, the previously gentle character of the Bench Trail begins to change as the canyon's topography requires the trail to go more radically up and down. After contouring around a ridge and crossing South Durham Creek, the route drops in a series of short, steep switchbacks to North Durham Creek (water, but no camps). The path then contours out to a ridge where a confusing ditch trail goes straight while the Bench Trail switchbacks to the left and drops to a junction. The road and the developed area visible on the Idaho side of the canyon are at Pittsburg Landing. The trail drops into Buckpasture Gulch before crossing yet another view-packed ridge and descending steeply to Pleasant Valley. Look for bears and some excellent campsites in this aptly named location.

Now the Bench Trail climbs gradually through a large meadow to a junction with the Snake River Trail. In a rugged detour around river-level cliffs, this lower trail has been forced to climb up to meet the Bench Trail at this point. The two trails follow the same route north for the next 2.8 miles.

Warning: *Beware of poison ivy in this section.*

After about 1.5 joyful ridge-and-meadow miles, the fun is over because the trail climbs a shadeless gully *steeply* to a pass. Take a well-deserved rest at the top to enjoy the great views in all directions. As the trail descends toward Somers Creek there are some fine views down to the river.

At a junction near the rounded summit called Englishman Hill, the Snake River Trail departs to the right while the Bench Trail makes a short jog left to Somers Creek at the site of burned down Somers Ranch. This is a fine spot for lunch or to camp for the night. After passing a junction with a trail to Somers Point, the Bench Trail climbs gradually up grassy slopes and through lush riparian areas to Hog Creek. Keep right at a junction and then cross some beautiful grassy terraces before dropping very steeply over loose, boot-skidding rocks to splashing Camp Creek (which, despite its name, has no decent flat spot to camp). Climb to a grassy saddle and then traverse an open terrace dotted with bushes on the way to inviting Tryon Creek Ranch. This ranch house and its outbuildings are still used by Forest Service crews, so the area is well maintained. A hose provides a steady flow of water from an unseen spring.

Tip: *If you have some extra energy in the evening, invest it in the fine side trip out to Tryon Viewpoint—0.6 mile northeast along the trail to Lookout Creek.*

From Tryon Creek Ranch the Bench Trail makes a long, wickedly steep 2000-foot climb to Tryon Saddle.

Tip: *Try to tackle this section in the shade of evening or the cool of the morning.*

Views from the windswept saddle are outstanding, especially of Deep Creek Canyon to the west. Elk populate the nearby slopes. Low-growing phlox and other flowers help to give this treeless pass an alpine feeling.

To continue your tour, keep right at the saddle, contour around a basin, and then begin the long descent to Deep Creek. This section of

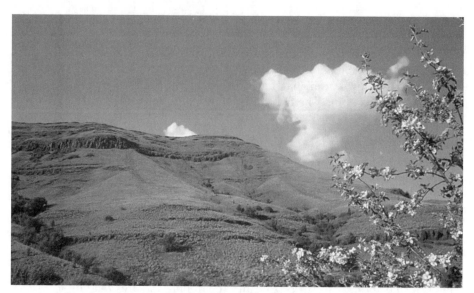

View from Tryon Creek Ranch

trail was elaborately rebuilt in 1998, so the previously steep descent is now much easier on the knees. The new route drops through a mix of rocky areas and trees before following a small creek for the final 0.5 mile. There is an excellent camp in the trees next to Deep Creek at the bottom of the descent.

The trail turns north and takes a joyful course as it follows the clear, rushing waters of Deep Creek. You pass through a surprisingly lush and shady forest of ponderosa pine, Douglas fir, grand fir, and mixed deciduous trees. The hiking is easy and beautiful through this environment, which is unusual for Hells Canyon—more closely resembling the higher-elevation forests of the Blue Mountains. Familiar forest residents like red-breasted nuthatches, porcupines, Douglas squirrels, and chipmunks find good habitat here. In early May look for huge serviceberry bushes, some as big as trees, putting on a showy display of white blossoms.

You pass the junction with a trail headed for Cow Creek before reaching a nice campsite. Continue straight to Deep Creek Ranch, which marks the end of the easy creekside forest walk. The immediate ranch area is reserved for the exclusive use of a commercial outfitter.

Tip: A little downstream from the ranch is a nice flat area where backpackers can make a comfortable camp.

You ford Deep Creek next to the ranch house and then begin to climb a mostly open slope above the cliffs lining lower Deep Creek's canyon. The climb tops out several hundred feet above Deep Creek Ranch, where there are terrific views of the lower canyon. Sadly, the trail now loses virtually all of that hard-won elevation as it drops to Little Deep Creek. There are good camps here, or rather there *would be* if the site weren't so badly churned to dust and made into a toilet by cattle. The smell, dust, and polluted stream are extremely upsetting, partly because this environmental damage is so unnecessary. At a minimum, areas where trails and streams cross should be fenced off to reduce this concentrated impact on the land and to preserve campsites.

The trail climbs gradually away from Little Deep Creek up an open grassy slope. Eventually you'll come to a fence line at a high pass where there are outstanding views. From this vantage point you can see all the way to Dug Bar Ranch, the end point of your hike. The path makes a long descent to Dug Creek and a junction with the trail to Lord Flat.

Warning: Beware of poison ivy near Dug Creek. The thickets here are the worst on the entire trip.

A short distance further is a second junction, this one with the Snake River Trail coming up from the right. Keep straight, climb a bit to reach a great view overlooking Dug Bar, and then drop steeply to the ranch. The well-marked public trail goes to the right around the ranch area.

Tip 1: Don't miss the short side trail to a sign discussing the Nez Perce Indians' crossing of the Snake River near here in 1877. While crossing the flooding river as they did is not advisable, it does feel great to jump in briefly, both to cool down and to wash off a few layers of dirt before hiking the last few hundred yards to your car.

Tip 2: Don't forget to allow plenty of time for the long, slow drive back out the Dug Bar Road to Imnaha.

POSSIBLE ITINERARY

	Camp	Miles	Elevation Gain
Day 1	Hat Creek	11.5	3700
Day 2	Temperance Creek	10.2	2100
Day 3	Kneeland Place	10.4	2300
Day 4	Tryon Creek Ranch	14.7	2800
Day 5	Little Deep Creek	9.3	2800
Day 6	Out	7.2	1200

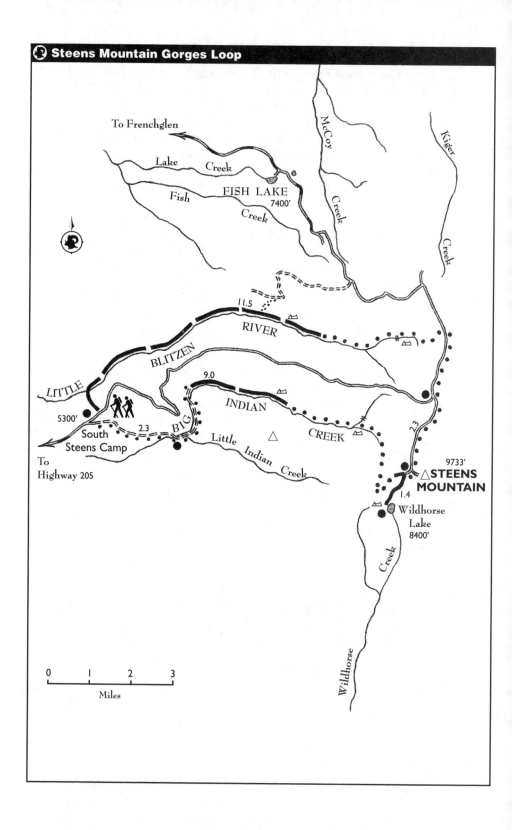

To Frenchglen

Lake Creek

Fish Creek

McCoy Creek

Kiger Creek

FISH LAKE
7400'

11.5

RIVER

BLITZEN

LITTLE

5300'

9.0

INDIAN

CREEK

South Steens Camp

2.3

BIG

Little Indian Creek

2.3

To Highway 205

9733'
△STEENS MOUNTAIN

1.4

Wildhorse Lake
8400'

Wildhorse Creek

0   1   2   3
Miles

27 Steens Mountain Gorges Loop

RATINGS (1–10)			MILES	ELEVATION GAIN	DAYS	SHUTTLE MILEAGE
Scenery	Solitude	Difficulty				
10	8	9	26	4200	2–4	N/A
			(28)	(5400)	(3–4)	

MAP USGS—*Fish Lake & Wildhorse Lake*

USUALLY OPEN Mid-June to October

BEST Late June/late September

PERMITS None

RULES Fires strongly discouraged

CONTACT Burns District, BLM, (541) 573-4400

SPECIAL ATTRACTIONS Solitude; incredible scenery; fall colors; wild-flowers

PROBLEMS Steep and very difficult scrambles up and down canyon headwalls; difficult stream crossings; thunderstorms; early season snowfields; limited shade; ticks (especially in spring and early summer); rattlesnakes

HOW TO GET THERE Drive south from Burns on Highway 205 for 60 miles to Frenchglen. Continue south on Highway 205 for another 9 miles to a well-marked gravel road going east. This is the southern end of the Steens Mountain Loop Road. Ominous signs here warn of possible blizzards. (When completely open, this is the highest road in Oregon, so they're not kidding.) Drive east on this decent gravel road for about 18 miles to Blitzen Crossing. About 2.5 miles beyond the bridge is the recently developed South Steens Campground. Turn into this campground and park near the marked trailhead.

INTRODUCTION Steens Mountain dominates the landscape of southeastern Oregon. At 9733 feet it towers over the hills and marshes of the surrounding desert, and can be seen for hundreds of miles in all directions.

People are drawn to this landmark for many reasons, not least of which is the scenery.

The majestic beauty of this desert mountain has no equal in Oregon or, arguably, anywhere else in North America. The cliffs on the mountain's eastern escarpment drop more than 5500 feet to the flat expanse of Alvord Desert. On the gently sloping west side of the mountain, ice age glaciers carved immense U-shaped gorges that are among the most impressive in the world. In most of North America, forests now obscure the evidence of past glaciation. Here, however, the only trees are scattered mountain mahogany and a few aspen groves near the bottom of canyons. Thus, the geologic history is spectacularly displayed for all to see. Waterfalls stream down steep walls that rise thousands of feet above the canyon floor. Clear, rushing streams flow through meadows sprinkled with wildflowers. Wildlife is plentiful, including bighorn sheep, badgers, coyotes, bobcats, and the occasional rattlesnake (especially in the lower parts of the canyons). Best of all, the isolation and the lack of official trails mean there's plenty of solitude—except, perhaps, during the fall hunting season. If you do this hike just before the higher parts of the loop road open to cars, you may have the entire trip to yourself. The road's lower elevations open in May.

Note 1: The snowpack on Steens Mountain is extremely variable. The highest parts of the loop road typically open around July 1; therefore,

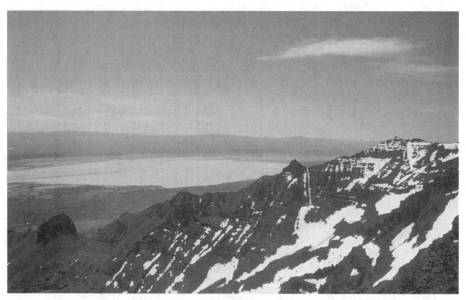

Alvord Desert and Steens Rim from the summit of Steens Mountain

the last week of June is ideal for this trip. Call ahead to the BLM office in Burns for the latest conditions.

Note 2: *Steens Mountain is a fragile island in a desert. Minimum impact techniques are especially critical here. Fires in particular should be avoided. The country is dry and wood is scarce, so bring a backpacking stove.*

DESCRIPTION Walk east to the small parking area for the family tenting section and pick up an old jeep track here. Follow this jeep track east as it gains elevation and then drops steeply to a berm, beyond which all vehicles (including bicycles) are prohibited. The route now crosses Indian Creek.

Warning: *In spring or early summer, this can be a cold and potentially difficult ford.*

Tip: *A sturdy walking stick and wading shoes will come in handy.*

On the opposite side, continue on the abandoned jeep track and quickly reach a crossing of Little Indian Creek (possibly wet but not a problem). This side creek flows down from its own scenic gorge—a worthwhile dayhike, if you have the time. Your route now goes north, following the main canyon of Big Indian Creek. Less than 1 mile beyond the first crossing is the second ford of the creek. This time the streambed is a bit wider so the crossing is easier.

The old road provides easy walking as it slowly gains elevation. Springs and small tributaries provide ample water early in summer. The mostly flat canyon bottom and the nearby stream mean that you can camp almost anywhere. The canyon turns east and grows ever more dramatic, with continuous and awe-inspiring views of the high peaks and cliffs. Sagebrush and juniper give way to more frequent meadows and occasional groves of aspen, and wildflowers become more numerous. Patches of snow from the previous winter add to the scenery.

Tip: *Photographers will need an extra-wide-angle lens to capture the enormity of this gorge.*

About halfway up the canyon the route fades out in a meadow. A large grove of aspen trees makes this a particularly inviting campsite. The road eventually disappears and a sketchy trail continues up the canyon. It is sometimes lost amidst sagebrush, aspens, or lush meadows, but the trail isn't really necessary. Be sure to look downstream from time to time to enjoy ever-improving views of this huge gorge. The relatively easy hiking ends at the sloping basin beneath the canyon headwall, one of Oregon's most spectacular locations. Flowers bloom in abundance, waterfalls cascade down the lava walls, and the surrounding cliffs rise almost 2,000 feet. There are plenty of possible campsites but not much shade.

Up to this point the going has been fairly easy, but sturdy boots and strong lungs are needed for the next section. Exiting the basin requires a steep uphill scramble over sometimes loose rocks. There is no single "best" route, but the recommended way is to turn south, following the left side of one of the creek's larger branches. Scramble up the grassy and rocky slopes toward the base of a pinnacle of pitted rock. You pass to the left of this pinnacle and soon reach a small upper basin where the going is easier. Continue to travel south over grassy alpine terraces to a saddle with a view of Little Wildhorse Lake, in the next drainage to the south. Turn left (east) and scramble past some rock outcroppings to a cliff-edge view of large Wildhorse Lake. This basin often remains snow covered into July, but later in the season the lake sits in a lovely meadow filled with wildflowers. Follow the ridgeline first north, then east around the head of this basin. As you approach the end of a spur road, a path leads down to Wildhorse Lake—a highly recommended side trip if the basin isn't filled with snow and ice.

Hike up the spur road for 0.2 mile to a road junction, where you should turn right for the short uphill side trip to the highest point on Steens Mountain. A radio tower and buildings intrude on the wilderness setting, but the view is amazing! Even the peaks of the Cascade Range are visible on clear days. Best of all, though, is the view east to the large, flat playa called Alvord Desert, over a vertical mile below.

Tip: Bring binoculars to look for bighorn sheep here and at other spots overlooking the eastern cliffs.

If the Steens Mountain Loop Road is not yet open to traffic, you should have this view all to yourself. The trade-off for solitude is the need to walk over some large snowfields.

Walk north along the summit spur road for 2.5 miles past a remarkable overlook of Big Indian Gorge to a junction with the main loop road. The high alpine grasslands in this area are alive with wildflowers in early August. Continue north along the road to the overlook of massive Little Blitzen Gorge.

Brace your knees because the next obstacle is a very steep scramble down the headwall cliffs of Little Blitzen Gorge. The cliffs directly below the overlook are ridiculously steep, so try the slopes either 0.5 mile farther north or about 0.3 mile south for a marginally easier route. It's about 1600 feet down to the floor of the canyon and there is no trail, so carefully pick your way down the rocky terrain. This effort is amply rewarded because the large, boggy basin below the headwall is only slightly less impressive than the one in Big Indian Gorge. Here you will enjoy more of the cliffs, wildflowers, clear streams, and generally outstanding scenery characteristic of Steens Mountain. There are numerous possible campsites to spend a night amidst this grandeur.

From the top of a small waterfall that drops from the headwall basin you'll enjoy a marvelous view down the canyon. Now a sketchy trail follows the north bank of the stream. This path is worth following because it improves and becomes a reasonably good trail as it continues downstream.

Your route travels past a second waterfall and through scenic meadows filled with grasses, wildflowers, and pungent sage. Near the creek aspens provide frames for photographs as well as welcome shade. Dark canyon walls rise in cliffs and columns on either side. About 4 miles down the canyon, a sketchy pack trail meets our route from the north. This little-used path switchbacks steeply up the north wall to a jeep track south of Fish Lake. The canyon floor is wide and nearly level near this junction, with several nice meadows and good campsites. A few old cabins and stock corrals add historical interest.

The Little Blitzen River Canyon slowly angles southwest as the stream's descent gets a bit steeper. The sage, mahogany trees, and brush get thicker at lower elevations, so views are somewhat limited for the rest of the way. After passing a massive buttress on the south wall, the river and the trail begin to angle a little more to the south before breaking out into the rolling sagebrush country at the mouth of the canyon. At a fence line, the trail turns left and fords the river.

Warning: *This crossing can be waist deep in early summer.*

The trail continues south, away from the river, as it climbs over a low ridge and gradually descends to the loop road at a signed trailhead. An easy 0.5-mile walk down the road leads back to your car and the close of an incredibly scenic trip.

POSSIBLE ITINERARY

	Camp	Miles	Elevation Gain
Day 1	Big Indian Gorge	8.3	1700
Day 2	Little Blitzen Gorge	9.0	3200
	(with side trips to Wildhorse		
	Lake and Steens summit)		
Day 3	Out	8.4	500

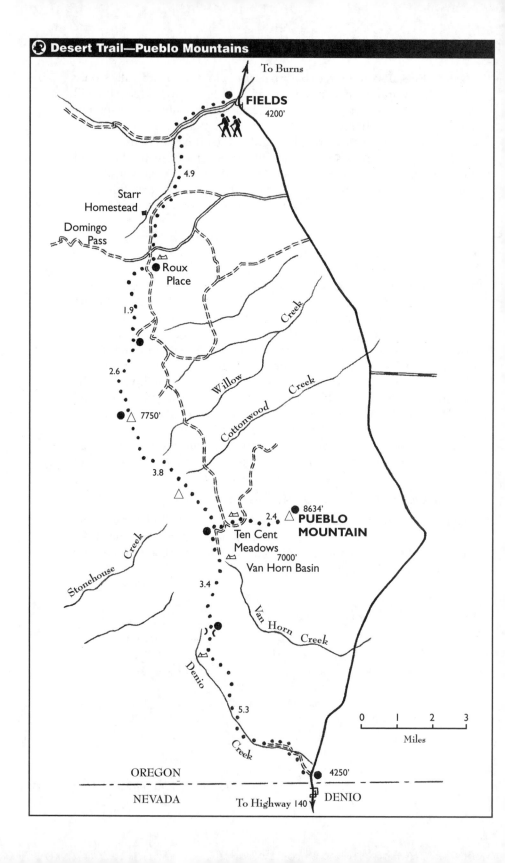

Desert Trail—Pueblo Mountains

To Burns

● **FIELDS**
4200'

4.9

Starr
Homestead

Domingo
Pass

● Roux
Place

1.9

2.6

△ 7750'

Willow   Creek

Cottonwood   Creek

3.8

△

2.4
△ ● 8634'
**PUEBLO
MOUNTAIN**

Ten Cent
Meadows

Stonehouse Creek

△ Van Horn Basin
7000'

Van Horn Creek

3.4

△

Denio

5.3

Creek

OREGON

NEVADA

To Highway 140

● 4250'

DENIO

0   1   2   3
Miles

28 Desert Trail–
Pueblo Mountains

RATINGS (1–10)			MILES	ELEVATION GAIN	DAYS	SHUTTLE MILEAGE
Scenery	Solitude	Difficulty				
8	9	7	22	6500	2–3	20
			(29)	(8200)	(3–4)	

MAP Desert Trail Association—*Pueblo Mountains Section*

USUALLY OPEN Mid-May to November

BEST Mid-June

PERMITS None

RULES Fires strongly discouraged

CONTACT Burns District, BLM, (541) 573-4400

SPECIAL ATTRACTIONS Expansive views; solitude; wildflowers

PROBLEMS   Route-finding difficulties; no shade; limited water; rattlesnakes

HOW TO GET THERE Both ends of this trip are on a good paved highway with an easy car shuttle between them—a real blessing in an area where road access is typically over poor dirt tracks. Start from the tiny town of Fields. To reach it, drive Highway 205 and a good county road for 120 miles south from Burns. The south trailhead is at Denio on the Oregon-Nevada border only 20 miles further south.

INTRODUCTION Until recently, almost no one in Oregon had heard of the Pueblo Mountains. If you told someone you were going to "the Pueblos," they assumed you were driving to the American Southwest to check out old Native American dwellings. Even today, despite a good paved road along their base and a segment of the Desert Trail running through them, the Pueblos remain isolated and receive relatively little use. But this desert range has a great deal to offer. Views seem to stretch to eternity. There are permanent streams and springs (rare for southeastern Oregon). Enough snow falls that the high cliffs and peaks are picturesquely streaked with white into June, and spring wildflowers put on a beautiful show. Don't expect much shade, however, as trees are limited to a few mountain mahogany and aspen.

The Desert Trail through this range is marked by large cairns that set only a general course through the terrain without a defined footpath. Hikers must pick their own way from one distant pile of rocks to the next.

> **Tip:** Bring a good map, a compass, and binoculars to help locate each cairn. The Desert Trail Association's map that includes compass bearings to each cairn is indispensable.

> **Warning:** In places magnetism in the rocks can throw off compass readings. Be careful you actually see the next cairn before proceeding.

DESCRIPTION   From the north end of "downtown" Fields (i.e., the single building that serves as store, post office, and gas station), hike 2 miles west on the McDade Ranch Road and then turn south at a cattle guard. Cross Williams "Creek" (probably dry) and follow a fence line for 0.5 mile. Head briefly west about 100 yards along another fence to reach a jeep road and once again turn south. Stick with this jeep road for about 2 miles (with a short detour around the Starr Homestead) to Domingo Pass Road. Shortly thereafter head southwest along a fence line. Follow this fence to its end, then continue southwest for about another 100 yards to a grove of aspens at the Roux Place Springs, the first reliable water.

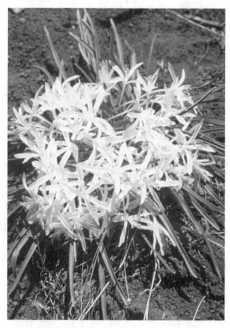

> **Note:** The springs are on private land. If you wish to camp, do so on public land, 200 yards or more to the south.

Continue south and contour at a roughly constant elevation around two hills to a jeep track that comes up from the east. Here you should find the first of the

Star of Bethlehem flower

series of cairns you'll be following for the remainder of this trip. Ahead is a long and difficult climb up a steep gully and hillside. Views to the north of distant Alvord Desert and Steens Mountain steadily improve as you climb. Closer at hand are the crags of the Pueblos as well as small flowers and colorful lichens on the rocks underfoot.

Warning: The route often crosses areas of loose rocks so exercise caution.

Tip: Be sure to check out an interesting rock with a large hole in it near cairn #7.

Reach the ridgecrest near cairn #8 and enjoy grand views in all directions—particularly to the west over the Rincon Valley and beyond. Stick with the up-and-down ridgecrest, often on game trails, to the top of a mountain. The bulk of your climbing is now complete, so congratulate yourself and enjoy the hard-won view. Reshoulder your pack and drop down the east side of the ridge. You pass a welcome spring and then contour around the cliffs above the head of Willow Creek.

Now you round a ridge at a saddle near cairn #22 and turn south. Towering cliffs rise to the west for the next 2 miles, and twisted mountain mahogany adds to the scenery. Cross a small tributary of Cottonwood Creek and then pass a grove of stunted aspen trees on the way to Ten Cent Meadows, set in a mile-wide saddle between the main ridge of the Pueblos on the west and hulking Pueblo Mountain on the east. There are possible campsites here, with nearby spring water.

You meet a jeep road coming up from Arizona Creek and follow it south for 1.2 miles as it drops into beautiful Van Horn Basin. There are many possible places to camp near Van Horn Creek, with aspen groves providing shade.

Tip 1: The morning view over the creek and the aspen groves of Van Horn Basin to the snow-streaked ridge of the Pueblos is a photographer's dream.

Tip 2: Don't miss the side trip from here to the summit of Pueblo Mountain. It's about 2.5 miles to the top and the route is often over steep and loose rocks, but the view is well worth the effort. There is, of course, no trail but you don't really need one.

To continue your tour, leave the jeep road at cairn #32 and climb, often steeply, up a sidehill. You walk along the top of a long rock ledge as the route works toward the pass between Van Horn and Denio basins. The views, as expected, are outstanding, especially to the east of massive Pueblo Mountain and of Van Horn Basin with its many aspen groves. After a well-deserved stop at the pass, proceed south into the Denio Creek drainage as you rapidly lose elevation. Wildflowers are particularly abundant here. At a large aspen grove there is room to make a pleasant camp beneath the trees, with nearby water.

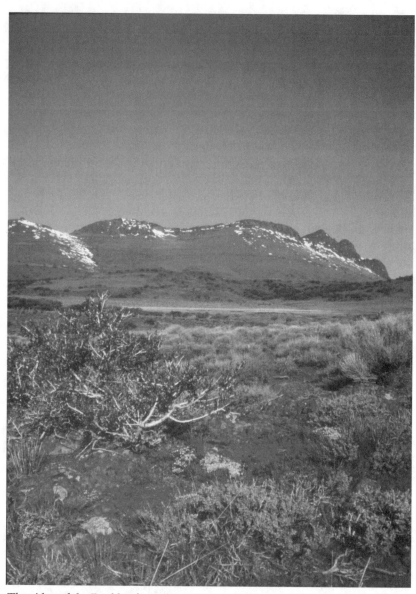

The ridge of the Pueblos from the east

Now the route makes a long, poorly marked detour to the east around a parcel of private land in Denio Basin. You cross a fence line marking the end of private property and meet a jeep road as you continue to descend the canyon of Denio Creek.

Tip: *Cattle trails through here are often confusing, but they provide easier walking through the sagebrush.*

Cross the creek a couple of times and then reach an interesting old stone cabin. For the final 1.8 miles the route follows a jeep road down to Denio.

POSSIBLE ITINERARY			
	Camp	Miles	Elevation Gain
Day 1	Roux Place Spring	5.2	1100
Day 2	Van Horn Basin	9.2	3600
Day 3	Denio Basin (with side trip up Pueblo Mountain)	9.5	3200
Day 4	Out	5.0	300

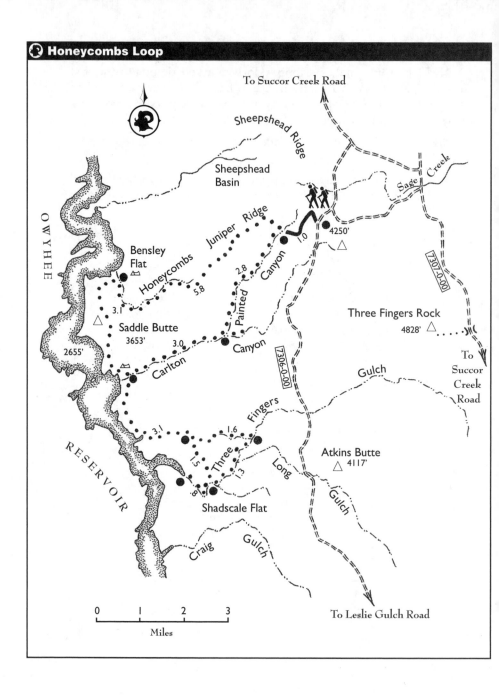

To Succor Creek Road

Sheepshead Ridge

Sheepshead Basin

Sage Creek

OWYHEE

Bensley Flat

Honeycombs

Juniper Ridge

Painted Canyon

4250'

7307-0-00

Three Fingers Rock
4828'

To Succor Creek Road

2.8

5.8

3.1

Saddle Butte
3653'

3.0

Canyon

Carlton

7306-0-00

Gulch

2655'

3.1

1.6

Fingers

Three

Long

Gulch

Atkins Butte
△ 4117'

1.5

1.3

RESERVOIR

.8

Shadscale Flat

Craig Gulch

Gulch

To Leslie Gulch Road

0   1   2   3
Miles

Honeycombs Loop

RATINGS (1–10)			MILES	ELEVATION GAIN	DAYS	SHUTTLE MILEAGE
Scenery	Solitude	Difficulty				
9	10	8	17	3500	2–3	N/A
			(29)	(6400)	(3–4)	

MAP USGS—*Three Fingers Rock & Pelican Point*

USUALLY OPEN April to November

BEST Early May/September

PERMITS None

RULES Fires strongly discouraged. Camping in Leslie Gulch is allowed only at Slocum Creek Campground.

CONTACT Vale District, BLM, (541) 473-3144

SPECIAL ATTRACTIONS Colorful rock formations; solitude

PROBLEMS Limited water; poor road access (or complicated boat transport); no trails; rugged hiking; rattlesnakes

HOW TO GET THERE For those without boat transportation, access to the closest roads is easier from the south. Drive north from Jordan Valley on Highway 95 for 18 miles, and turn left on gravel Succor Creek Road. Follow this route for about 13 miles (or 3.5 miles north of the well-marked Leslie Gulch turnoff) and turn left onto McIntyre Spring Road. The driving difficulties start here. With mud, rocks, and little or no maintenance, this road will never be mistaken for a super highway. On the positive side, the drive provides wonderful views of cliff-edged McIntyre Ridge and the chance to see wild horses.

Drive over a saddle about 1 mile east of prominent Three Fingers Rock (well worth the relatively short walk to explore) and continue north another 3.5 miles. Turn left in a grassy little valley holding Sage Creek, which is dry by early summer. This road, even worse than the one you've been on, climbs about 2.4 miles to a junction.

> *Tip: If this road is too rough, an alternate approach is to continue north from Sage Creek for 0.3 mile and then turn left on Road 7307-0-00 for*

2 miles. Turn south on Road 7306-0-00 for 1.8 miles to the previously mentioned junction with the road up Sage Creek.

In a low pass 0.4 mile south of this junction, park beside a livestock watering tank.

INTRODUCTION Tucked away on the east side of Owyhee Reservoir is a land of striking beauty. In the dry canyons of this desert country is a collection of oddly shaped rock pinnacles, towers, and cliffs painted in a colorful array of browns, reds, and oranges. In spring, especially after a wet winter, the sagebrush and grasses turn green, and wildflowers like balsamroot and paintbrush add yellows, reds, and other colors to the scene. Hikers familiar with the canyonlands of southern Utah will feel right at home.

Actually getting there, however, is not easy. A good gravel road goes down Leslie Gulch, so this canyon has become popular with hikers, photographers, and other admirers. Stretched out to the north are several equally spectacular canyons whose remoteness provides much more solitude. For the backpacker, the best access is either by boat from Owyhee Reservoir or over rough and poorly marked dirt roads that are torture on cars. The boat access requires finding someone willing to shuttle you down the reservoir about 25 miles to Bensley Flat and then return to pick you up after your trip. There is no commercial service and relatively few private boaters go this far down the lake. As for the roads, after it rains, only high-clearance four-wheel-drive vehicles should try them. One option is to park on one of the area's

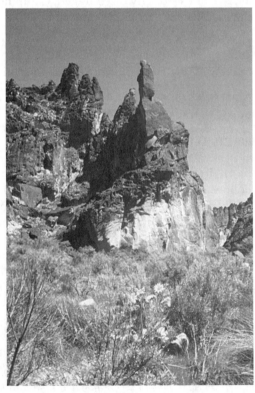

The Honeycombs in Carlton Canyon

good roads (through Leslie Gulch or Succor Creek Canyon) and then take a mountain bike to the starting point for your hike.

Warning: Water ranges from scarce to nonexistent. The only reliable year-round source is Owyhee Reservoir, and this should be treated with both chemicals and filtering before drinking. On the other hand, beware of occasional thunderstorms that may cause flash floods.

DESCRIPTION   Having survived the drive, strap on a pair of sturdy boots (good ankle support is essential in this steep, rocky, trailless terrain) and head northwest on a jeep track. You top a low hill and then turn south and drop to a gully at the head of Painted Canyon. Hike down this ravine as it grows narrower and more spectacular. In places you may be forced to make rugged detours around cliffs and dry waterfalls.

Tip: Bring a rope to lower your pack over especially steep and dangerous sections before climbing down yourself.

The long, steep descent ends as the canyon bottom widens and levels out. Multicolored cliffs and spires rise on both sides, and as you continue down the canyon the geologic scenery does nothing but improve. Near the mouth of Painted Canyon the walls narrow considerably before breaking out into Carlton Canyon.

Tip: To see more towers and cliffs drop your pack and explore east into upper Carlton Canyon for 0.5 mile.

Turning west, you'll find the scenery remains good, although not as continuously dramatic as Painted Canyon.

Tip: After about 1 mile look for a side canyon to the north that is well worth exploring.

About 2 miles from Painted Canyon and 1 mile from the mouth of Carlton Canyon, you'll reach some high buttresses on either side that are especially dramatic. You can make camp in the flats where the canyon widens near Owyhee Reservoir—just don't count on any shade.

You can make an excellent but rugged day trip to Three Fingers Gulch from a base camp at the mouth of Carlton Canyon. Pack some water and hike south along the up-and-down slopes beside Owyhee Reservoir. After about 2 miles cross the mouth of a good-sized canyon and then climb up this canyon's south ridge for 1.5 miles to where it levels out. From here you turn south up a second ridge bordered on the west by cliffs and pinnacles.

Note: These cliffs go steeply down to the reservoir, which explains why you had to make this detour. Access beside the water is not feasible.)

Descend east to a saddle, then *carefully* scramble down a *very* steep and narrow gully between two cliffs. You should reach the base of Three Fingers Gulch near a fork in the canyon at Shadscale Flat where a very faint jeep road approaches from the south. Be sure to explore downstream through this scenic, narrow gulch to the Owyhee Reservoir.

Warning: The last 0.2 mile to the reservoir requires some tough scrambling.

Tip: If you're really ambitious, scramble up the canyon's steep south slope to enjoy cliff-top views of Three Fingers Gulch. Once on top, turn west for about 0.5 mile to reach the terrific views atop the impressive cliffs rising directly from the waters of Owyhee Reservoir.

Turning east (up-canyon), keep left at the forks where you entered Three Fingers Gulch and travel between two impressive cliffs. After about 0.8 mile you'll reach the mouth of Long Gulch at a point distinguished by a tall pinnacle. Keep left, following Three Fingers Gulch, and 0.3 mile later turn left again into a small canyon. You can climb this canyon all the way to the top of the ridge you came in on earlier in the day and retrace your route back to Carlton Canyon.

To complete the recommended backpack loop, go north from the mouth of Carlton Canyon along the sagebrush-covered hills beside Owyhee Reservoir. After about 1 mile you'll reach the base of Saddle

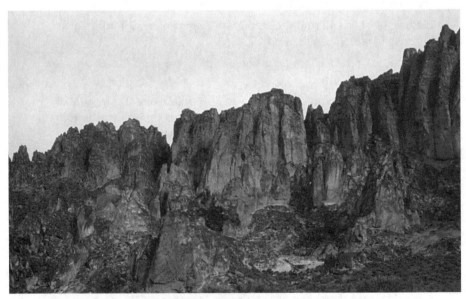

The Honeycombs from Bensley Flat

Butte. Scramble over the pass on the east side of this landmark and then drop down a ravine to the large expanse of Bensley Flat. You can comfortably camp almost anywhere on this bench. There are even a few boaters' cabins and willow trees near the reservoir's shore.

Tall reddish-brown cliffs rise to the east of Bensley Flat.

Tip: These cliffs are best photographed in the low light of late evening.

From the south end of the cliffs, you walk up a scenic draw that heads initially south and then loops around to the northeast. This gulch goes through the heart of the "Honeycombs"—a spectacular region with a dizzying display of colorful rock formations, many pockmarked with holes and small caves. The north side of the canyon is particularly impressive.

About 2 miles from the canyon's mouth you pass to the left of a large rock monolith and then continue to follow the canyon bottom as it climbs and turns east. At the head of the canyon, scramble very steeply to the right to reach the top of long, rolling Juniper Ridge, where the walking is much easier as you follow game and cattle trails.

Warning: The crisscrossing trails along this ridge can be confusing. The correct route follows a generally northeast course along the top of this wide ridge.

After about 2 miles turn east, drop down a gully, and look for the jeep track coming down to the head of Painted Canyon.

Tip: If Juniper Ridge reaches a little saddle and starts to climb moderately steeply toward a 4500-foot highpoint, then you have gone about 0.5 mile past the proper turnoff.

Pick up the jeep route and follow it back to your vehicle (either car or bicycle).

POSSIBLE ITINERARY

	Camp	Miles	Elevation Gain
Day 1	Mouth of Carlton Canyon	6.8	200
Day 2	Mouth of Carlton Canyon (day trip to Three Fingers Gulch)	12.0	2900
Day 3	Out (via Honeycombs)	9.9	3300

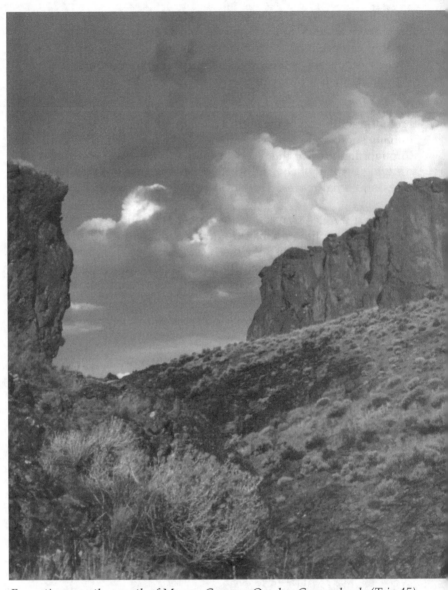

Formation near the mouth of Massey Canyon, Owyhee Canyonlands (Trip 45)

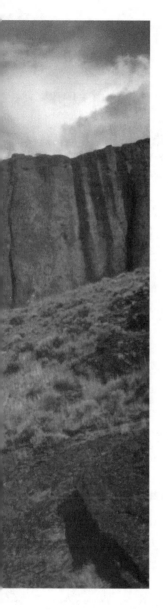

Other Backpacking Options

Although this book includes what the author considers to be the *best* long backpacking trips in Oregon, there are many other options for the adventurous backpacker. With some creativity and a good set of contour maps, a backpacker could easily spend a lifetime in this diverse state.

What follows is an overview of some additional recommended trips, with just enough description to whet the appetite. Since many of these hikes are in lesser-known areas, they are excellent options for solitude lovers. (Unless specifically noted, none of these trips requires a permit.)

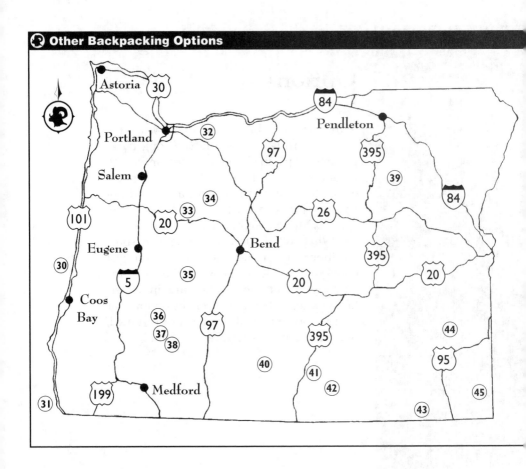

30 Oregon Dunes Loop

RATINGS (1–10)			MILES	DAYS
Scenery	Solitude	Difficulty		
7	3–8	5	Varies	Varies

MAP USFS—*Oregon Dunes National Recreation Area*

USUALLY OPEN All year

BEST Winter/mid-May

SPECIAL ATTRACTIONS Extensive sand dunes

PROBLEMS Summer crowds; quicksand in winter

Although this area is crowded in summer, it is blessedly quiet in winter. Mid-May features blooming rhododendrons in the forests. There are several options for backpackers, but your best choice is some combination of beach and inland dune hiking south from the Siltcoos River, past Tahkenitch Creek, to Umpqua Spit, and back.

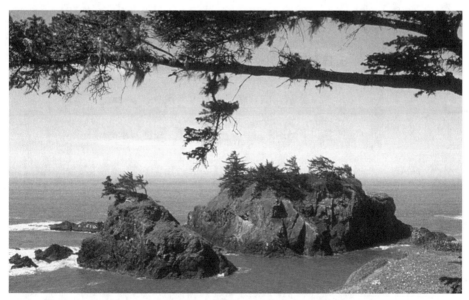

Rocks near Thunder Rock in Samuel Boardman State Park (Trip 31)

31 South Coast

RATINGS (1–10)			MILES	DAYS
Scenery	Solitude	Difficulty		
10	4	5	Varies	Varies

MAP   Use *100 Oregon Coast & Coast Range Hikes* book

USUALLY OPEN   All Year

BEST   Mid-April to May

SPECIAL ATTRACTIONS   Spectacular coastal scenery

PROBLEMS   Very limited camping options; some road walking

Between Gold Beach and Brookings, the Oregon coast is at its most spectacular. By connecting beach walks with trail segments, a *stunningly* scenic hike is possible. Lack of campsites, proximity to the highway, and sometimes crowded trails make this area more popular with dayhikers than backpackers. Hike north from Brookings through Samuel Boardman State Park as far as time and ambition allow. Two possible stopping points are Arch Rock and Cape Sebastian.

32 Talapus Trail

RATINGS (1–10)			MILES	DAYS
Scenery	Solitude	Difficulty		
7	6	9	38	4–6

MAP   USFS—*Trails of the Columbia Gorge*

USUALLY OPEN   Late May to October

BEST   June to mid-July

SPECIAL ATTRACTIONS   Solitude; views

PROBLEMS   Rugged up-and-down route; irregular trail maintenance

For those who want to explore the rugged backcountry of the Columbia River Gorge, the Talapus Trail is perfect. This exhausting hike connects several trails as it traces a circuitous inland route along ridges, through forests, in and out of steep canyons, and past numerous viewpoints. Start in the west at Larch Mountain and end in the east below Mount Defiance. Excellent side trips include Nesmith Point, Wauneka Point, Tanner Butte, and Tomlike Mountain.

33 Old Cascades Loop

RATINGS (1–10)			MILES	DAYS
Scenery	Solitude	Difficulty		
4	9	5	42	4–5

MAP None really adequate (try the latest district map)

USUALLY OPEN June to November

BEST Late June to July

SPECIAL ATTRACTIONS Solitude; old-growth forests

PROBLEMS New trail that's not yet on maps; limited views

The star attraction of this recently completed route is the old-growth forest. Several sloping wildflower meadows and ridgetop viewpoints add variety and scenic interest. You start from the Maude Creek Trailhead, reached by following Road 2067 off Highway 20 west of its junction with Highway 22. Climb over Crescent Mountain and the Three Pyramids and then loop counterclockwise via Scar Mountain, Knob Rock, Donaca Lake, and Pyramid Creek back to Crescent Mountain and your car.

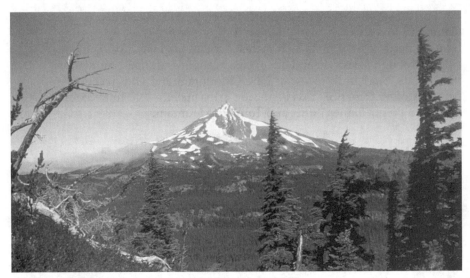

Mount Jefferson from Sugar Pine Mountain

34 Table Lake Loop

RATINGS (1–10)			MILES	DAYS
Scenery	Solitude	Difficulty		
9	5	7	25+	3–5

MAP Geographics—*Mount Jefferson*

USUALLY OPEN Mid-July to October

BEST Late July to August

SPECIAL ATTRACTIONS Diverse volcanic scenery; great views

PROBLEMS Mosquitoes

This hike tours the scenic east part of the Mount Jefferson Wilderness. The route includes many outstanding views, a lava flow, lakes, and plenty of room for exploring. Start from the Jefferson Creek Trailhead, reached from the lower Metolius River near Sisters, and follow the Jefferson Creek Trail to Table Lake.

Tip: Schedule extra time for spectacular dayhikes to The Table and Hole-in-the-Wall Park.

Return by the Sugar Pine Ridge Trail to the south. Permits are required.

Warning: The lower and middle elevations in the eastern half of this area were badly burned in the 2003 B&B Fire. Expect a blackened landscape for several years.

35 Waldo Lake Loop

RATINGS (1–10)			MILES	DAYS
Scenery	Solitude	Difficulty		
6	5	3	21+	2–6

MAP   USFS—*Waldo Lake Wilderness and Recreation Area*

USUALLY OPEN   Mid-June to late October

BEST   Mid-August to September

SPECIAL ATTRACTIONS   Easy trail; good swimming; scenic lake vistas; huckleberries

PROBLEMS   Mosquitoes (through early August); poor fishing (the lake is too pure to support many fish)

Large, beautiful, and incredibly clear Waldo Lake is the only major lake in Oregon with a shoreline trail good for backpackers. (Other lakes all have too many roads, people, and/or speed boats.) In addition to having pleasant scenery, the loop trail is also relatively easy, making this trip ideal for families with children. Excellent side trips to places like Black Meadows, Waldo Mountain Lookout, the Eddeeleo Lakes, and the Rigdon Lakes are fine for those looking for more exercise. The lake is north of Highway 58 east of Oakridge.

36 North Umpqua River

RATINGS (1–10)			MILES	DAYS
Scenery	Solitude	Difficulty		
7	6	3	Varies	Varies

MAP USFS—*Umpqua National Forest*

USUALLY OPEN March to November

BEST April and May

SPECIAL ATTRACTIONS Whitewater rafters; beautiful river and canyon scenery; wildlife; waterfalls; fishing

PROBLEMS Poison oak; nearby major highway

The relatively new North Umpqua Trail follows the beautiful North Umpqua River from Idleyld Park all the way to its source. Even though the trail parallels busy Highway 138, it has a surprisingly wild character. A series of bridges and road crossings allow for one-way trips of 5 to 70 miles. The best early-season choice is the section from Idleyld Park to Toketee Lake—a distance of 47 miles. The upper part of this trail is described in Trip 13.

37 Rogue-Umpqua Divide

RATINGS (1–10)			MILES	DAYS
Scenery	Solitude	Difficulty		
7	7	5	27	3

MAP USFS—*Rogue-Umpqua Divide Wilderness*

USUALLY OPEN Late May to November

BEST Mid- to late June

SPECIAL ATTRACTIONS Wildflowers; rock formations; views; solitude

PROBLEMS Long car shuttle

This little-known wilderness is a pleasant surprise to most Oregon hikers. There are meadows filled with a stunning array of wildflowers, subalpine lakes, fascinating rock formations, and expansive views. The best tour of the area starts in the south at a pass on gravel Road 68 northwest of Prospect. Hike north past Abbott Butte, Elephant Head, Anderson Butte, and Hershberger Mountain.

Tip: Don't miss the short side trip to the Hershberger Lookout.

Continue along spectacular Rocky Ridge, descend to Fish Lake, and exit at the Fish Lake Creek Trailhead off Road 2840 in Umpqua National Forest. Side trips abound.

38 Upper Rogue River

RATINGS (1–10)			MILES	DAYS
Scenery	Solitude	Difficulty		
6	4	3	Varies	Varies

MAP USFS—*Rogue River National Forest*

USUALLY OPEN Late May to November

BEST Late October

SPECIAL ATTRACTIONS Beautiful river and canyon scenery; fall colors; waterfalls

PROBLEMS Some crowded areas; nearby major highway

Even though it's never far from a busy highway, this long river path is a real treat. While a few of the more geologically interesting attractions, such as the Natural Bridge, are crowded with tourists, other areas are quiet. Late October brings few people and exceptional fall colors. Start from the Crater Rim viewpoint along Highway 238 west of Diamond Lake and hike downstream past waterfalls, campgrounds, and through attractive old-growth forests all the way to Prospect (48 miles). Numerous access points allow for shorter options.

39 North Fork John Day River

RATINGS (1–10)			MILES	DAYS
Scenery	Solitude	Difficulty		
6	8	4	25	3–6

MAP   USFS—*North Fork John Day Wilderness*

USUALLY OPEN   June to November

BEST   June to October

SPECIAL ATTRACTIONS   Excellent fishing; canyon scenery

PROBLEMS   Some burned areas

This forested canyon hike is especially appealing to anglers. Opportunities to try your luck in the rushing waters of the North Fork John Day River are found around every bend. Several historic old cabins are also interesting. For a one-way downhill hike, start from the North Fork Trailhead along paved Road 73 northwest of Sumpter. The trail stays close to the stream's north bank for its entire length. The lower trailhead is on dirt Road 5506, most easily reached from Ukiah to the west.

40 Fremont Trail

RATINGS (1–10)			MILES	DAYS
Scenery	Solitude	Difficulty		
7	10	5	Varies	Varies

MAP   USFS—*Fremont National Forest*

USUALLY OPEN   Mid-June to November

BEST   Late June to July

SPECIAL ATTRACTIONS   Views; solitude; bighorn sheep

PROBLEMS   Limited water in places

Fremont National Forest is developing an excellent new long trail that connects nearly all parts of this little known but scenic forest. Currently about 90 percent complete, this trail explores the high peaks of the Warner Mountains, travels along a remote ridge west of Valley Falls, crosses the Chewaucan River, and then follows Winter Ridge for views of Summer Lake. Eventually plans call for the trail to connect all the way west to the Pacific Crest Trail and east to the Desert Trail. Early summer provides the best conditions when seasonal water sources are available and the area supports lots of wildflowers.

Abert Rim

RATINGS (1–10)			MILES	DAYS
Scenery	Solitude	Difficulty		
9	10	7	24	3

MAP USGS—*Little Honey Creek & Lake Abert South*

USUALLY OPEN June to November

BEST June

SPECIAL ATTRACTIONS Bighorn sheep; views!

PROBLEMS No trail; almost no water

Abert Rim is the tallest and perhaps the most impressive fault scarp in the world. An extended backpacking trip is the ideal way to appreciate the enormity of this scenic rim. Off Highway 140 northeast of Lakeview, go north on Road 3615 and then dirt Road 377 to the Abert Rim overlook. Walk cross-country north along the view-packed rim's edge. Exit either at Mule Lake (poor road access) or via the steep use path down to Highway 395 at Poison Creek.

42 Hart Mountain–Poker Jim Ridge

RATINGS (1–10)			MILES	DAYS
Scenery	Solitude	Difficulty		
8	10	8	30	3

MAP USGS—*Hart Lake, Warner Peak, Campbell Lake & Bluejoint Lake East*

USUALLY OPEN Mid-May to November

BEST June

SPECIAL ATTRACTIONS Wildlife; views; solitude

PROBLEMS Poor road access; no trails; rugged route; ticks; very limited water

This is a long but very scenic hike along Hart Mountain's desert escarpment. From Plush (northeast of Lakeview) drive south along the rough, narrow, dirt track beside Hart Lake's east shore for about 4 miles and park. You start with a difficult scramble up to the high plateau of Hart Mountain. Turn north to Warner Peak and Rock Creek and then cross the refuge access road and continue along Poker Jim Ridge to the recommended exit at Bluejoint Lake. Wildlife and views are abundant throughout. Except for Rock Creek, water is nonexistent. Permits are required.

43   Trout Creek Mountains Loop

RATINGS (1–10)			MILES	DAYS
Scenery	Solitude	Difficulty		
8	9	8	44	4–6

MAP   USGS—*Doolittle Creek & Little Whitehorse Creek*

USUALLY OPEN   Mid-May to October

BEST   June/early October

SPECIAL ATTRACTIONS   Solitude; fishing; wildlife; fall colors (especially aspens); wildflowers

PROBLEMS   Poor roads; no trails; private land to circumvent

These little-known desert mountains near the Nevada border are a real treat for hikers. Since the area has recently been managed to restrict cattle, the streams and wildflowers are in good shape. One of several possible trips is a long loop hike that starts near privately owned Sweeney Ranch and goes up scenic Whitehorse Creek Canyon. Turn west along a jeep road on the high ridge of the Trout Creeks and then return via Little Whitehorse Creek Canyon.

44   Lower Owyhee Canyon Rim

RATINGS (1–10)			MILES	DAYS
Scenery	Solitude	Difficulty		
9	10	6	40	3–5

MAP   USGS—*Lambert Rocks & Rinehart Canyon*

USUALLY OPEN   April to November

BEST   May

SPECIAL ATTRACTIONS   Wildlife; magnificent canyon scenery

PROBLEMS   Awful road access; very limited water; poison ivy near the river; rattlesnakes

The *best* way to experience the wild and scenic canyon of the Owyhee River is to float the stream. The *next* best way is to backpack the rim—a highly rewarding adventure, despite the lack of trails.

Warning: *The "roads" here are passable only to high-clearance four-wheel-drive vehicles.*

From the tiny community of Rome, go northwest on gravel and then dirt county roads through a private ranch (leave all gates the way you found them) to the start of public land near Crooked Creek. Park and walk east and then north along the canyon rim.

Tip: *Don't miss exploring Chalk Basin, and the side trip to the amazing view from Iron Point.*

Exit at the Rinehart Canyon "road" (more of a jeep track) northwest of Jackson Hole.

45 Louse Canyon

RATINGS (1–10)			MILES	DAYS
Scenery	Solitude	Difficulty		
8	10	10	50	4–7

MAP   USGS—*Rawhide Springs, Drummond Basin & Three Forks*

USUALLY OPEN   May to October

BEST   September

SPECIAL ATTRACTIONS   Solitude; desert canyon scenery

PROBLEMS   Poor road access; very rough scrambling required; rattlesnakes; lots of wading (or even swimming)

This is an *extremely* remote and rugged hike down the canyon of the West Little Owyhee River. The canyon features towering cliffs, colonnades and pinnacles, pools of water reflecting canyon walls, and wildlife. The hike is *extraordinarily* rough and should be contemplated only by very experienced and well-equipped hikers willing to expend an enormous amount of both physical and mental energy to enjoy this adventure. Start from Anderson Crossing at the mouth of Massey Canyon and end near Three Forks—both reached by very poor dirt roads. Good maps are essential.

Index

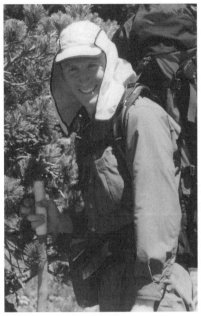

Photo by Becky Lovejoy

ABOUT THE AUTHOR

Douglas Lorain's family moved to the Pacific Northwest in 1969, and he has been obsessively hitting the trails of his home region ever since. With the good fortune to grow up in an outdoor-oriented family, he has vivid memories of countless camping, hiking, birdwatching, and other trips in every corner of this spectacular area. Over the years he calculates that he has logged well over 30,000 trail miles in this corner of the continent, and despite a history that includes being bitten by a rattlesnake, shot at by a hunter, charged by grizzly bears (twice!), and donating countless gallons of blood to "invertebrate vampires," he happily sees no end in sight.

Lorain is a photographer and recipient of the National Outdoor Book Award. His books cover only the best trips from the thousands of hikes and backpacking trips he has taken throughout Washington, Oregon, and Idaho. His photographs have been featured in numerous magazines, calendars, and books, and his other guidebook titles include *100 Classic Hikes in Oregon, Afoot & Afield Portland/Vancouver, Backpacking Idaho, Backpacking Washington, Backpacking Wyoming,* and *One Night Wilderness: Portland.*

Although he considers his real home to be on the trail, those few days he is forced to spend indoors, he lives in Portland, Oregon, with his wife, Becky Lovejoy.